Nutrition and Diet Re

PHYTOCHEMICALS FOR THE CONTROL OF HUMAN APPETITE AND BODY WEIGHT

NUTRITION AND DIET RESEARCH PROGRESS

Diet Quality of Americans
Nancy Cole and Mary Kay Fox (Authors)
2009. 978-1-60692-777-9

School Nutrition and Children
Thomas J. Baxter (Editor)
2009. 978-1-60692-891-2

Appetite and Nutritional Assessment
Shane J. Ellsworth and Reece C. Schuster (Editors)
2009. 978-1-60741-085-0

**Beta Carotene: Dietary Sources,
Cancer and Cognition**
Leiv Haugen and Terje Bjornson (Editors)
2009. 978-1-60741-611-1

**Flavonoids: Biosynthesis, Biological
Effects and Dietary Sources**
Raymond B. Keller (Editor)
2009. 978-1-60741-622-7

**Handbook of Vitamin C Research:
Daily Requirements, Dietary Sources and Adverse Effects**
Hubert Kucharski and Julek Zajac (Editors)
2009. 978-1-60741-874-0

Diet Quality of Americans
Nancy Cole and Mary Kay Fox (Authors)
2009. 978-1-60876-499-0

Supercritical Fluid Technology Applied to the Manufacture of Prebiotic Carbohydrates
Tiziana Fornari, Fernando Montañés, Agustín Olano and Elena Ibáñez (Authors)
2010. 978-1-60876-978-0

Biological Effects of β -Carotene
Rosa Martha Perez Gutierrez, Adriana Maria Neira Gonzalez and Sandra Lugardo Diaz (Authors)
2010. 978-1-61668-609-3

Nutritional Education
Ida R. Laidyth (Editor)
2010. 978-1-60876-078-7

Dietary Supplements: Primer and FDA Oversight
Timothy H. Riley (Editor)
2010. 978-1-60741-891-7

Handbook of Nutritional Biochemistry: Genomics, Metabolomics and Food Supply
Sondre Haugen and Simen Meijer (Editors)
2010. 978-1-60741-916-7

Dietary Fiber, Fruit and Vegetable Consumption and Health
Friedrich Klein and Georg Möller (Editors)
2010. 978-1-60876-025-1

Biological Effects of β -Carotene
Rosa Martha Perez Gutierrez, Adriana Maria Neira Gonzalez, Sandra Lugardo Diaz (Authors)
2010. 978-1-61668-256-9

Maintaining a Healthy Diet
Anna R. Bernstein (Editor)
2010. 978-1-60741-856-6

Nutritional Factors and Osteoporosis Prevention
Masayoshi Yamaguchi (Author)
2010. 978-1-60876-929-2

Vitamin D: Biochemistry, Nutrition and Roles
William J. Stackhouse (Editor)
2010. 978-1-61668-273-6

**Phytochemicals for the Control of Human
Appetite and Body Weight**
S.A. Tucci, E.J. Boyland and J.C. Halford (Authors)
2010. 978-1-61668-676-5

Vitamin D: Biochemistry, Nutrition and Roles
William J. Stackhouse (Editor)
2010. 978-1-61668-713-7

**Phytochemicals for the Control of Human
Appetite and Body Weight**
S.A. Tucci, E.J. Boyland and J.C. Halford (Authors)
2010. 978-1-61668-897-4

Vitamin D: Biochemistry, Nutrition and Roles
William J. Stackhouse (Editor)
2010. 978-1-61668-713-7

**Phytochemicals for the Control of Human
Appetite and Body Weight**
S.A. Tucci, E.J. Boyland and J.C. Halford (Authors)
2010. 978-1-61668-897-4

Nutrition and Diet Research Progress

PHYTOCHEMICALS FOR THE CONTROL OF HUMAN APPETITE AND BODY WEIGHT

S.A. TUCCI, E.J. BOYLAND AND J.C. HALFORD

Nova Science Publishers, Inc.
New York

For permission to use material from this book please contact us:
Telephone 631-231-7269; Fax 631-231-8175
Web Site: http://www.novapublishers.com

NOTICE TO THE READER

The Publisher has taken reasonable care in the preparation of this book, but makes no expressed or implied warranty of any kind and assumes no responsibility for any errors or omissions. No liability is assumed for incidental or consequential damages in connection with or arising out of information contained in this book. The Publisher shall not be liable for any special, consequential, or exemplary damages resulting, in whole or in part, from the readers' use of, or reliance upon, this material.

Independent verification should be sought for any data, advice or recommendations contained in this book. In addition, no responsibility is assumed by the publisher for any injury and/or damage to persons or property arising from any methods, products, instructions, ideas or otherwise contained in this publication.

This publication is designed to provide accurate and authoritative information with regard to the subject matter covered herein. It is sold with the clear understanding that the Publisher is not engaged in rendering legal or any other professional services. If legal or any other expert assistance is required, the services of a competent person should be sought. FROM A DECLARATION OF PARTICIPANTS JOINTLY ADOPTED BY A COMMITTEE OF THE AMERICAN BAR ASSOCIATION AND A COMMITTEE OF PUBLISHERS.

LIBRARY OF CONGRESS CATALOGING-IN-PUBLICATION DATA

Available upon Request
ISBN: 978-1-61668-676-5

Published by Nova Science Publishers, Inc. ⏶ *New York*

CONTENTS

Preface   ix

Abbreviations   1

Chapter 1   Introduction   3

Chapter 2   Mechanisms that Regulate Body Weight   7

Chapter 3   Phytochemicals and Weight Control   11

Chapter 4   Conclusion   33

References   43

Index   73

PREFACE

The regulation of energy balance and body weight is under the influence of complex neural, metabolic and genetic interactions. Despite this, obesity is now a global epidemic associated with significant morbidity and mortality in adults and ill health in children. Thus the effective management of obesity has become an important clinical issue. To date there are very few approaches to weight management effective in the long term. This contrasts with disorders such as anorexia and bulimia nervosa which also appear in part to be phenomena of the modern environment and equally difficult to treat. This book will focus on the mechanisms of body weight regulation and the effect of plants or plant extracts (phytochemicals) on these mechanisms. As phytochemicals are often not single compounds but rather a mixture of different unrelated molecules, their mechanism of action usually targets several systems. In addition, since some cellular receptors tend to be widely distributed, sometimes a single molecule can have a widespread effect. We will attempt to describe the main phytochemicals that have been suggested to affect the homeostatic mechanisms that regulate, and some non-homeostatic system that influence, body weight. The in vitro, pre-clinical and clinical data will be summarised and scientific evidence will be reviewed.

ABBREVIATIONS

2-AG	2-arachodonoyl glycerol
5-HT	Serotonin, 5-Hydroxytryptamine
α-MSH	α- Melanocyte-stimulating hormone
Δ^9-THC	Δ^9-Tetrahydrocannabinol
A	Adrenaline
ARC	Arcuate nucleus
ATP	Adenosine-triphosphate
BMI	Body mass index
CART	Cocaine-and-amphetamine-regulated transcript
CCK	Cholecystokinin
CNS	Central nervous system
COMT	Catechol-o-methyl transferase
CPT	Carnitine palmitoyltransferase
CRH	Corticotropin releasing hormone
DA	Dopamine
DMN	Dorsomedial nucleus
EC	Epicatechin
ECG	Epicatechin gallate
EE	Energy expenditure
EGC	Epigallocatechin
EGCG	Epigallocatechin gallate
EI	Energy intake
FFA	Free fatty acids
GALP	Galanin-like peptide
GI	Gastrointestinal
GLP-1	Glucagon-like peptide-1

GCBE	Green coffee bean extract
GTE	Green tea extract
HCA	(−)- hydroxycitric acid
LH	Lateral hypothalamus
NA	Noradrenaline
NPY	Neuropeptide Y
PFC	Prefrontal cortex
PVN	Paraventricular nucleus
PYY	Peptide YY
TG	Triglycerides
SNS	Sympathetic nervous system
UCP-1	Uncoupling protein 1
VTA	Ventral tegmental area

Chapter 1

INTRODUCTION

Ingestive behaviour in humans is influenced by a complex set of innate and cognate processes modulated by culture and the external environment [1]. From the physiological point of view, an appropriate supply of micro- and macronutrients is required for life. This has lead to the evolution of strong biological mechanisms that defend food supply just as they do for other biological needs [2]. Eating more food than necessary for daily energy expenditure (EE) in times of food plenty increased chances of survival during subsequent periods of famine. As a consequence, most vertebrates developed the ability to store a considerable amount of energy and some micronutrients for later use. However, this ability has now become one of the biggest health risks for many human populations [1]. The uninterrupted supply of cheap energy-dense foods together with an increasingly sedentary lifestyle has led to obesity in a large segment of the human population.

Weight gain and obesity are a result of positive energy balance due to a long-term mismatch between energy intake (EI) and EE. Obesity constitutes a major global health problem as it is a risk factor for several chronic disorders such as diabetes, hyperlipidemia, hypertension, cardiovascular disease, osteoarthritis and some forms of cancer [3]. The most widely advocated means of resolving the obesity epidemic are changes in lifestyle, dieting and exercise. Nevertheless, while losing weight in the short term is achievable, data suggest that maintaining reduced body weight over the long term has proven to be exceedingly difficult for most people [4, 5]. At least part of the reason behind the difficulty of maintaining a reduced body weight is the body's ability to activate adaptive mechanisms that act to minimize weight loss such as an increase in both the motivation to find food and the size of individual meals

[6] which is accompanied by a decrease in metabolic rate [7] that lasts until energy stores are replenished. Therefore one rationale for pharmacotherapy and alternative approaches has been to sustain weight loss behaviour by dampening these compensatory mechanisms. Pharmacologic agents designed to suppress hunger have promoted weight loss, but were often accompanied by unacceptable side effects. For instance, amphetamine-based anorexigens have been effective in some patients, but in some also produced a variety of undesirable effects of mood and behavioural expression. These agents are also prone to abuse and may have the potential to produce chemical dependency [8].

Nonetheless, over the last 20 years, many drugs lacking amphetamine-like side effects have been successfully employed. Some of these agents were the beta-phenethylamine derivatives which had lower abuse potential and proved to be useful in some individuals. Nevertheless, side effects such as insomnia, anxiety and irritability precluded its widespread use [8]. The limited efficacy of beta-phenethylamine derivatives prompted research into a new class of agents, ones acting on serotonergic neurotransmission. Fenfluramine hydrochloride (Pondimin[R]) and then dexfenfluramine hydrochloride (Redux[R], Adifax[R]) although widely effective, they were implicated in the development of cardiac valvulopathy [9] and in consequence withdrawn from the market. In 1997, sibutramine (Reductil[R], Meridia[R]), a serotonin (5-hydroxytryptamine; 5 -HT)-and noradrenaline (NA)-reuptake inhibitor was introduced into the market. Sibutramine possesses effective weight loss and low weight maintenance properties. However, its use has been associated with several psychiatric [10-14] and possible cardiovascular disorders related to transient increases in blood pressure and heart rate [15]. This may preclude its use in patients with particular psychiatric conditions (although the drug was originally developed as an anti-depressant [16]) and more importantly its effects on patients with cardiovascular conditions is still under investigation [17, 18]. Since such conditions are usually concomitant with obesity, potentially a proportion of obese patients may not be suitable for sibutramine therapy [19]. Orlistat (Xenical[R]), an intestinal lipase inhibitor, hinders the breakdown of fat in the intestines and as a consequence this undigested fat is not absorbed but excreted [20]. The presence of undigested fat in the bowels causes side effects (such as diarrhoea, abdominal pain, oily stools and faecal spotting) that limit use of orlistat [21]. Additionally, chronic gastrointestinal (GI) ailments like irritable bowel syndrome are clear contraindications for its use. These issues, along with the potential for abuse of this drug as a purgative, and possible deficiencies in fat soluble vitamins associated with use, have caused some concern. Nonetheless, a half dose of orlistat (Alli® , 60mg rather than 120 mg three times daily) has been approved in Australasia, USA and EU for over-the-counter use [21]. More recently, an approach that attempts to manipulate the mechanisms involved in the motivation to eat and the rewarding or hedonic properties of food is emerging. The drugs recently under investigation target the cannabinoid system which is thought to modulate food intake and energy balance.

Chapter 2

MECHANISMS THAT REGULATE BODY WEIGHT

SIGNALS OF ENERGY INTAKE AND FAT STORAGE

One of the major determinants of the survival of higher organisms including mammals is the ability to maintain a stable body weight. Body weight regulation mainly concerns adipose tissue since protein and carbohydrate stores in adults only vary a relatively small amount. Therefore, a chronic imbalance between EI and EE results in changes in adipose tissue mass [22]. Body weight, similarly to other physiological processes, is regulated by a feedback mechanism that integrates peripheral and central signals in order to generate an adequate response.

The afferent limb of the feedback mechanism of body weight regulation consists of substances that reflect the metabolic status of the organism. For instance, adipose tissue produces leptin. Leptin is the product of the *ob* gene [23] and correlates positively with the amount of adiposity [24]. Leptin levels are monitored by the hypothalamus, where the binding of leptin to its receptor alters the expression of several genes that encode for neuropeptides involved in modulating food intake and EE [25]. As with leptin, circulating levels of insulin are also proportional to adiposity [26]. Adiponectin is another protein produced by adipose tissue; similarly to leptin, its secretion depends on fat store status but in contrast to leptin adiponectin plays a fundamental role in promoting lipolysis. Adiponectin plasma concentration is inversely correlated with adiposity and increases after food restriction [27]. Ghrelin is the first described GI hormone that stimulates food intake [28], it is released by the stomach and the intestine in the fasting state and situations of anticipated eating. It is suspected that the high levels of ghrelin generated by low calorie diets could be responsible for rebound weight gain [29, 30]. Cholecystokinin (CCK) is synthesised by endocrine cells in the duodenum and jejunum, and it was the first gut hormone shown to dose-dependently decrease food intake in several species, including humans [31-33]. CCK is one of the earliest short-term satiety signals. Similarly to CCK, peptide YY (PYY) and glucagon-like peptide 1 (GLP-1) also have satiating properties, being released by the ileum and colon in response to the presence of lipids and carbohydrates.

CENTRAL CONTROL OF ENERGY BALANCE

The detection and integration of the above mentioned orexigenic and anorexigenic signals (reviewed in [34]) occurs in the hypothalamus. Due to the absence of a blood-brain barrier, the arcuate nucleus (ARC) of the hypothalamus is considered to play a key integrative role between the initial afferent signals from the periphery and the central nervous system (CNS) responses. In addition to expressing receptors for the above mentioned peripheral signals [35, 36], ARC neurones also sense blood glucose levels [37]. The ARC has neuronal subpopulations that produce orexigenic (neuropeptide Y (NPY) and agouti-related peptide (AgRP)) as well as anorexigenic peptides (α-melanocyte-stimulating hormone (α-MSH), galanin-like peptide (GALP), and cocaine-and-amphetamine-regulated transcript (CART)). The ARC neurones project to "second-order" neurones implicated in the control of feeding such as the paraventricular nucleus of the hypothalamus (PVN), the dorsomedial hypothalamic nucleus (DMN), and the lateral hypothalamic area (LH) [38, 39]. When adiposity signals reach the ARC, anorexigenic peptides are released which activate a catabolic circuit. In contrast, when adiposity signal concentrations in the brain are low, orexigenic peptides are released activating an anabolic pathway [40].

Initially the LH was identified as a 'hunger centre' because lesions in this area produced temporary aphagia, adipsia, and reductions in body weight. Two sets of neurones that contain either orexin [41] or melanin concentrating hormone [42], both potent stimulators of food intake, have been identified in this area. Both types of neurones have a wide projection field to key cortical, limbic, and basal forebrain areas [43, 44]. The DMN receives inputs from cells in the ARC and from brainstem centres. Lesions restricted to the DMH typically result in hypophagia. The PVN integrates signals of different brain regions and triggers endocrine (through corticotropin-releasing hormone (CRH) and thyrotropin-releasing hormone), and autonomic responses .

Another system, the endocannabinoid system, has recently been implicated in the regulation of appetite. The role of this system in feeding regulation is supported by reports indicating that endocannabinoid systems are essential to suckling and growth in neonates [45], and are involved in feeding responses across the phylogenetic scale [46]. Brain endocannabinoid levels have been reported to be elevated in fasted rats [47], and administration of cannabinoid receptor agonists increase food intake [48, 49] while antagonists decrease it [50]. Overall, current data indicate that tonic endocannabinoid release may be crucial to the normal expression of feeding and possibly to the long-term regulation of body weight. In addition, the biosynthesis of the endocannabinoids anandamide and 2-arachodonoyl glycerol (2-AG) appears to be regulated by leptin [51]. Thus, leptin administration suppresses hypothalamic endocannabinoid levels in normal rats; while genetically obese, chronically hyperphagic rodents express elevated, leptin-reversible, hypothalamic anandamide or 2-AG levels [52].

In addition to receiving a fairly complex input on the individual's metabolic status, the hypothalamus integrates the motivation and emotion-related features of feeding behaviour (via direct interactions with medial prefrontal (PFC) and cingulate cortex, basal forebrain and medial septal nuclei) with more fundamental aspects of appetitive and aversive responses (via interaction with nucleus accumbens (NAc), amygdala, ventral tegmental area (VTA), substantia nigra and raphe) [53-58]. After processing this information it sends its output mainly through three pathways: the endocrine system (pituitary gland), the sympathetic nervous system (SNS), and motor expression (promotion or inhibition of food intake) [59, 60]. These pathways constitute the efferent loop in the body weight control system. The endocrine system and SNS act mainly to control EE.

SYSTEMS IMPLICATED IN ENERGY EXPENDITURE

EE is the second aspect of energy balance (the first being food intake). Total EE is the sum of resting EE, the thermic effect of food, and EE related to activity (for review, see [61, 62]). Resting EE or basal metabolic rate is the energy used for cell metabolism to keep cells alive. The intrinsic inefficiency of these cellular events generates a certain amount of heat known as "obligatory thermogenesis". In humans, resting EE is relatively fixed, it primarily reflects body weight and composition, and is generally the largest component of total energy expenditure (65–75%) [63]. In addition, warm-blooded animals need to generate additional heat to reach the optimal core body temperature, also known as "adaptive thermogenesis." [64]. Since energy consumption during thermogenesis can involve oxidation of lipid fuel molecules, regulation of thermogenesis in response to metabolic signals can also contribute to energy balance and regulation of body adipose stores [65].

Food intake is associated with stimulation of EE, also known as diet-induced thermogenesis or the thermic effect of food. The magnitude of the thermic effect is 5 to 10% of the caloric content of ingested carbohydrates, 0 to 3% of that for lipids and 20 to 30% of that for proteins and is, in a situation of energy balance, approximately 10% of the daily energy intake [66]. This energy is consumed during intestinal absorption of nutrients, the initial steps of their metabolism in the body and their storage. In addition, when food is ingested, homeostatic mechanisms need to be activated in order to digest, absorb, distribute and store the nutrients as quickly as possible. The SNS plays a crucial role in this response, since it regulates postprandial blood flow distribution, blood pressure and thermogenic responses to a meal [67]. The SNS role in postprandial thermogenesis depends on the size and macronutrient composition of the meal and is most evident after high carbohydrate meals [68]. Obesity leads to increased levels of sympathetic activity, and overconsumption and high carbohydrate diets may lead to gradual downregulation of the β-adrenoceptor-mediated thermogenic and metabolic responses, which may be involved in the development of obesity [69-71].

In lean and obese adults weight loss significantly reduces EE beyond levels predicted solely on the basis of changes in weight and body composition [72]. However, there is little evidence of energy wastage in periods of overnutrition [73, 74]. Small increases in EE, if not accompanied by an equivalent increase in EI, would induce a slight negative energy balance and thereby influence body weight regulation in the long term. Thus, direct stimulation of EE may be used as a strategy to improve body weight loss and prevent (re)gain. It is well established that increasing EE at the same time as decreasing EI is more likely to result in significant weight loss and more importantly, weight loss maintenance.

Chapter 3

PHYTOCHEMICALS AND WEIGHT CONTROL

When considering the mechanisms responsible for body weight maintenance it can be concluded that it could be achieved through manipulation of the following: EE (mainly thermogenesis), appetite suppression/satiety enhancement, and fat and glucose absorption blocking. The phytochemicals described below can alter either one single component but more frequently they exert their effect through a combination of modes of action.

Foods are an obvious source of phytochemicals and many may possess specific ingredients that alter appetite beyond the effects expected by normal nutrient loads. Additionally, many therapeutic herbs and nutrients have far fewer side effects and may provide an alternative treatment or could be used to enhance the effect of prescription medications. In this chapter, recent *in vitro*, animal and human studies on the effects of phytochemicals in body weight are examined and summarised. Although most phytochemicals that affect body weight regulation have a complex mechanism of action, for the purpose of this book they will be grouped according to their main effect (increase or decrease body weight) and the site of main mechanism of action (CNS, peripheral or both).

PHYTOCHEMICALS THAT DECREASE
BODY WEIGHT MAINLY THROUGH
A PERIPHERAL MECHANISM

Korean Pine Nut Oil

Nuts, in their various forms, are widely consumed across the globe, and have recently been linked with the positive health benefits of the Mediterranean diet [75]. Nut consumption is purported to have many health benefits, particularly some protective effects against cardiovascular disease [76, 77] , and it has also been suggested that nuts have satiety enhancing ingredients as there is some epidemiological evidence linking nut consumption inversely with body weight [77]. These properties may relate to their general nutritional content such fibre and protein and/or specific oils. Oils are major constituents of nuts, constituting as much as 60% of the total weight in pine nuts.

Korean pine nut oil (Pinnothin®) is obtained by natural pressing of Korean pine nuts (*P. koraiensis*) and it contains triglycerides (TG) and more than 92% poly- and mono-unsaturated fatty acids (PUFAs and MUFAs) like pinolenic acid (C18:3), linoleic acid (C18:2) and oleic acid (C18:1) [78]. Korean Pine nut oil is claimed to be unique in that it contains approximately 15% pinolenic acid (C18:3). Previous studies on Korean pine nut oil have shown beneficial effects on lipoprotein metabolism and immune function [79, 80]. *In vitro*, Korean pine nut free fatty acids (FFA) have the ability to significantly increase the release of satiety hormones such as CCK from the murine neuroendocrine tumour cell line STC-1 [81]. *In vivo*, fat digestion leads to formation of monoglycerides and fatty acids. These products of fat digestion lead to an increase in CCK, GLP-1 and PYY secretion. However, only fatty acids with chain lengths $\geq$ C12 are capable of triggering the release of CCK and GLP-1 [82, 83]. Moreover, CCK delays gastric emptying and produces a subsequent increased feeling of satiety and a decreased appetite. In terms of inducing satiety hormone secretion, long chain fatty acids are more effective than medium chain fatty acids, and poly-unsaturated fatty acids are more effective than mono-unsaturated fatty acids [84, 85].

The fact that Korean pine nut FFA had the ability to significantly increase satiety hormones *in vitro* lead to the examination of this potential effect in human participants. Administration of pine nut FFA to overweight postmenopausal women produced a significant increase of CCK-8 and GLP-1 without altering ghrelin or PYY levels. In addition, Korean pine nut FFA also lowered the appetite sensation "prospective food intake" and "desire to eat", importantly, these effects lasted up to 4 hours [81, 86]. Another study showed that Korean pine nut FFA (2 grams) produced a significant 9% reduction in ad-libitum food intake thirty minutes after dosing compared with the placebo control. No differences between PinnoThin® and the placebo were seen at the evening meal, suggesting that there is no compensation for the lesser food intake during lunch [87]. Importantly, the studies performed so far report no adverse effect of the compound either during the study period or at post study debriefing. Whether Korean pine nut FFA produce beneficial effects on appetite and body weight beyond that of similar FFA remains to be demonstrated. Certainly, since there are other oil based satiety enhancing ingredients on the market, it could be possible to determine if these effects are due to distinct phytochemical components or are generic to these types of dietary lipids.

Palm Oil + Oat Oil Fractions

Olibra® is a fat emulsion formulated from palm oil (40%) and oat oil fractions (2.5%). Olibra® has a similar mechanism of action to that of Korean pine nut oil. This is an increased and prolonged release of PYY, CCK and GLP-1 [88, 89] that inhibits upper gut motility (to slow gastric emptying and intestinal transit) which generates an indirect satiety effect [90, 91].

Compared to other functional foods and phytochemicals, the evidence supporting the effects of this product on appetite is more comprehensive. Double-blind, placebo-controlled reports indicate that Olibra® administration to lean, overweight and obese individuals significantly decreased energy and macronutrient intake up to 36 h post-consumption [88, 92]. It also reduced hunger and desire to eat [93]. The chronic effects of Olibra® were investigated in a double-blind, placebo-controlled study where it was administered during a weight loss and weight maintenance scheme [89]. The results of this study suggest that Olibra® administration could help to maintain weight after weight loss programmes. Taken together these findings indicate that in addition to having acute effects on EI and hunger/satiety, Olibra® could be beneficial for weight maintenance.

Gallic Acid

Gallic acid is an organic acid mainly found in gallnuts, sumac, witch hazel, tea leaves and oak bark. Gallic acid, the major hydrolytic product of tannic acid, it is also found free [94]. In rodents, administration of both tannic and gallic acid reduces food intake [95-97]. Initially it was thought that the reduction in food intake was mediated through taste aversion, however, later it was demonstrated that intravenous and intraperitoneal infusion of gallic acid also reduced intake which indicates that the mechanism of action of this compound involves more than sensory or GI factors [94]. However, studies performed in humans have not replicated effects found in rodents [97].

It has been hypothesised that gallic acid competes with catecholamines for inactivation via the enzyme catechol-o-methyl transferase (COMT). This enzyme inactivates catecholamines such as NA and adrenaline (A) [98] whose administration into rats results in anorexia [99]. In addition, recent studies have shown that gallic acid inhibits squalene epoxidase (SE), an enzyme involved in cholesterol synthesis [100] altering lipid metabolism [101].

Garcinia Cambogia

G. cambogia (Commercially available as (−)- hydroxycitric acid (HCA) extract from G. cambogia: Super CitriMax® HCA-SXS (HCA-SX®)) is a tree indigenous to southeast Asia. The active component is in its small fruit, also known as Malabar tamarind. The dried and cured pericarp of the fruit of this species contains up to 30% by weight of HCA [102]. These pericarp rinds have been used for centuries in regional cooking practices and are reported to make meals more filling and satisfying [103, 104] without any reported harmful effects. Clinical studies with HCA have encountered some mild adverse events such as headache, and upper respiratory tract and GI symptoms [105].

Administration of HCA to rats and mice suppresses appetite and body fat accumulation [106-111]. These effects are also evident in animal models of genetic obesity such as Zucker rats [112], however the effects in these rats seem to be only achieved when toxic doses are given [113]. Studies performed in humans have provided conflicting results. Several randomized placebo-controlled, single-blinded cross-over trials have shown that administration of HCA (1.2-1.5 g/day) to overweight participants did not produce any significant decrease in body weight or appetite variables [105, 114]. On the other hand, a laboratory based study with a similar design reported that daily administration of a relatively low dose of HCA (900 mg/day) over 2 weeks, although only producing minor changes in body weight, reduced EI in and sustained satiety [115]. In an 8 week study Preuss et al [116] found that 2,800 mg/day of HCA produced a reduction of 5.4% and 5.2% in baseline body weight and BMI respectively compared to controls. In addition, food intake, total cholesterol, LDL, TG and serum leptin levels were significantly reduced, while HDL levels and excretion of urinary fat metabolites (a biomarker of fat oxidation) significantly increased.

HCA may promote weight reduction through suppressed de novo fatty acid synthesis, increased lipid oxidation and reduced food intake [117]. Enhanced satiety may also account for the reported suppression of energy consumption but this has yet to be demonstrated. One potential mechanism accounting for the satiety effect of HCA involves the inhibition of adenosine-triphosphate (ATP) -citrate lyase, the enzyme that converts excess glucose into fat [118, 119]. Furthermore, by inhibiting ATP-citrate lyase, HCA reduces the availability of acetyl-CoA, the building block for fat synthesis. As a result, carbohydrates and fatty acids that would have become fat are diverted to glycogen synthesis. This metabolic change may send a signal to the brain that results in reduced appetite, reduced food intake and a decreased desire for sweets [107, 108]. A second possible mechanism for the anorectic effect of HCA is via acetyl CoA. By reducing acetyl CoA, malonyl CoA levels are reduced too. This decreases the negative feedback on carnitine acyltransferase [117] which leads to increased lipid transport into the mitochondria and inefficient oxidation with resultant ketone body formation. Ketones are purported appetite suppressants, however, several groups have failed to observe an association between ketosis and reported hunger level [120, 121]. Several additional mechanisms of action of HCA have been proposed, one report showed that HCA administration decreased body weight by increasing EE [110], however, the mechanism responsible for this effect has not been elucidated. A recent study demonstrated that HCA alters the expression of genes associated with adipogenesis such as PPARγ2, SREBP1c, C/EBPα, and aP2 as well as other visceral obesity-related biomarkers [111].

The conclusion arising from studies in humans provides some support for the claim that HCA may be more effective at moderating weight gain [122] than at promoting weight loss, making the compound potentially more useful for weight maintenance after an initial loss. Again more clinical data are needed.

PHYTOCHEMICALS THAT BLOCK PANCREATIC LIPASE AND ALPHA-AMYLASE

Currently, malabsorptive surgery is one of the most effective treatments for obesity [123], therefore it is not surprising that non-surgical approaches have focused on drugs that inhibit the absorption of macronutrients. Acarbose, an inhibitor of carbohydrate absorption, has been shown to have modest efficacy in the treatment of diabetes, but does not cause weight loss [124]. Dietary fat is the most energy dense macronutrient, and most closely linked to overweight and obesity. Therefore, the blockage of fat absorption is a logical target for an anti-obesity drug. The phytochemicals described below act by blocking the breakdown and consequent absorption of dietary carbohydrates and/or lipids.

Salix Matsudana

S. matsudana (Chinese willow) (one ingredient of Rev Hardcore® and Methyl Ripped®) is a species of willow native to north western China. Its leaves have been used for more than 3000 years in traditional Chinese medicine for the treatment of several ailments. It has recently been reported that the polyphenol extracts of *S. matsudana* have anti-obesity actions [125, 126]. In this study, oral administration of polyphenol fractions to dietary-induced obese mice reduced adiposity and body weight. *In vitro* analysis revealed that *S. matsudana* extract enhanced NA-induced lipolysis and inhibited the enzyme α-amylase which is involved in the digestion and absorption of carbohydrates. In addition, the polyphenol fractions also had an effect on lipid absorption since its presence completely inhibited the intestinal absorption of palmitic acid which is a product of oil hydrolysis. These results conclude that the effects *S. matsudana* are mainly due to the inhibition of carbohydrate and lipid absorption, and the acceleration of fat mobilisation through enhancement of NA-induced lipolysis in adipocytes [125]. Although *S. matsudana* extracts have been shown to have anti-obesity actions *in vitro* and in rodents, research in humans, especially on the long term effects, is lacking.

Platycodi Radix

Platycodi radix is the root of *Platycodon grandiflorum* A. DC (*Campanulaceae*), commonly known as Doraji (Chinese drug, 'Jiegeng', and Japanese name, 'Kikyo'). It has been used as a traditional oriental medicine, as extracts have been reported to have wide-ranging health benefits [127]. In some Asian cultures Platycodi radix is used as a food and employed as a remedy for adult diseases including hypercholesterolemia and hyperlipidemia [128].

Platycodin saponins are the primary constituents of Platycodi Radix [129]. Similarly to ginseng, the anti-obesity and hypolipidemic properties of Platycodin saponins are due at least in part to an inhibition of pancreatic lipase [130, 131]. Nevertheless, a study by Zhao et al [132] found that in rats, the decrease in body weight correlated with decrease in caloric intake, an effect not obviously attributable to lipase inhibition. They ascribed this effect to the ability of Platycodin saponins to reduce gastric secretion [133] , which in turn would cause a reduction in gastric digestion ability, generating food intake restriction. These results suggest that Platycodin saponins could be a potential therapeutic alternative in the treatment of obesity and hyperlipidemia [130, 131]. However, further data showing replication of these effects in humans are needed.

Kochia Scoparia

K. scoparia is a shrub whose fruits have been used in traditional Japanese and Chinese medicine, and also as food garnish in Japanese-style dishes [134]. There are several reports showing that in animals, the alcohol extract and saponins isolated from the fruit of *K. scoparia* inhibit blood glucose level increases through inhibition of glucose uptake in the small intestine [178-180], however, the exact mechanism responsible for this effect has not been elucidated. In addition, saponins from *K. scoparia* inhibit pancreatic lipase. The oral administration of a saponin rich fraction significantly suppressed the increases in body and adipose tissue weights in dietary-induced obese mice [134]. However, human clinical data are lacking.

Aesculus Turbinata

A. turbinata is a medicinal plant widely distributed in northwestern China. Its dried ripe seeds have been used as a carminative, stomachic, and analgesic for the treatment of distension and pain in the chest and abdomen [135]. The saponins extracted from the seeds are called escins. Recently, escins have been reported to show inhibitory effects on both the elevation of blood glucose levels [136] and pancreatic lipase activity in mice [137, 138] but there are no data regarding these effects in humans.

Tea Saponins

Three kinds of tea: oolong, green, and black, are widely used as traditional healthy drinks all over the world. Among the three teas, green and oolong tea have been traditionally reported to have anti-obesity and hypolipidemic actions. Black tea also contains many active ingredients [139], however some of these may not survive processing. These teas contain several different active ingredients.

Oolong Tea

Catechins in oolong tea are reported to prevent dietary-induced obesity by inhibiting small-intestine micelle formation [140], limiting the absorption of sugars by inhibiting α- glucosidase activity [141]. In dietary-induced obese mice, oolong tea catechins suppressed increases in body weight, parametrial adipose tissue weights, and adipose cell size by delaying the intestinal absorption of dietary fat through the inhibition of pancreatic lipase activity [139]. In a double-blind, placebo-controlled study, twelve weeks daily administration of oolong tea (containing 690 mg of catechins) to normal and overweight males (with daily EI set at 90%) produced a significant reduction in body weight (1.5%), body mass index (BMI) (1.5%), waist circumference (2.0%), and body fat mass (3.7%), compared to the placebo group [142]. These results suggest that oolong tea catechin consumption might be useful as an adjuvant during weight loss programmes.

Green Tea

In Asia, green tea is a widely consumed beverage and for centuries has been thought to possess significant health promoting effects [143]. The long term consumption of green tea and its extract (GTE) (commercially available as pills, patches, gums, mints, extracts, and ice creams) have been associated with weight loss mainly through a thermogenic mechanism [144]. It is particularly the catechins from the flavanols fraction of green tea which have received a lot of attention. Green tea is derived from drying and steaming the fresh tea leaves and thus no oxidation occurs, resulting in high levels of catechins. In contrast, black tea undergoes a full fermentation stage before drying and steaming [145] which lowers levels of catechins. The main active ingredients in GTE, the catechins epigallocatechin gallate (EGCG; Teavigo®), epigallocatechin (EGC), epicatechin gallate (ECG), and epicatechin (EC) are responsible for many of the beneficial effects of green tea [146, 147].

In vitro data suggest that the anti-obesity effects of green tea are at least partially mediated via inhibition of adipocyte differentiation and proliferation [148-150]. There is also evidence that green tea could reduce glucose and fat absorption by inhibiting GI enzymes involved in nutrient digestion [151, 152] . In addition, EGCG directly inhibits COMT, an enzyme that inactivates NA, thus prolonging the action of sympathetically released NA [153, 154]. GTE is also rich in caffeine which is a potent amplifier of thermogenesis when given in conjunction with other SNS agonists such as ephedrine, nicotine, catechins or capsaicin from chillies [155-159].

Studies have shown that green tea reduces adipose tissue weight in rodent models of obesity. These effects appear to be mediated via increased EE and decreased glucose uptake by skeletal muscle and adipose tissue respectively [160-162]. In humans the majority of studies that investigated the effects of GTE administration showed a significant decrease in body weight and body fat when compared to baseline. Body weight changes (corrected for changes in placebo group) ranged from 0.6 to −1.25 kg, whereas the change in body fat ranged from 0.5 to −1.8 kg [163-168]. However, it is important to highlight that in some of these studies participants were also subjected to moderate energy restriction (90% of individual energy requirements) [142, 169] or exercise [168]. In an open, uncontrolled study (not blinded and lacking a control group) administration of GTE to overweight participants produced a 4.6% decrease in body weight compared to baseline [170]. Nevertheless the majority of these studies were not strictly controlled for EI and physical activity. However, when food intake was monitored, there was no significant difference in EI between groups. Therefore it has been suggested that thermogenesis and fat oxidation are the main mechanisms responsible for weight loss [171-173]. Catechins from GTE have been associated with an increase in SNS activity, thermogenesis and fat oxidation in humans [142, 171].

A number of *in vitro*, pre-clinical and clinical studies were, and are currently being performed to investigate the anti-obesity effects of green tea. As of today, a body of evidence has accumulated, which scientifically supports the traditional notion that green tea reduces body weight by "eliminating fat". The results from preclinical and clinical studies strongly suggest that GTE, rich in catechins and caffeine, is an effective potentiator of sympathetically mediated thermogenesis and could be used as an adjuvant in the management of obesity [174]. Certainly the effects of GTE on weight control are worthy of further clinical investigation.

Green Coffee Bean

Green coffee bean extract (GCBE) (Quest Green Coffee [®], Svetol[®]) contains 10% caffeine and 27% chlorogenic acid as the principal constituents. The roasting process of coffee drastically reduces the level of chlorogenic acid and its related compounds [175]. Chlorogenic acid is a polyphenolic compound with antioxidative activity which has been reported to have a hypotensive effect [176] and to selectively inhibit hepatic glucose-6-phosphatase [177], which is a rate-limiting enzyme involved in gluconeogenesis. Administration of GCBE or chlorogenic acid to mice has a suppressive effect on weight gain and visceral fat accumulation [178]. Moreover, chlorogenic acid also reduces the level of hepatic TG. Interestingly, this effect is more potent than that of GCBE.

Carnitine palmitoyltransferase (CPT) is a rate-limiting enzyme that catalyses the transportation of metabolised and fatty acid to liver mitochondria for β-oxidation. GCBE administration enhances CPT activity [178]. However, CPT activity does not seem to be affected when caffeine and chlorogenic acid are administered separately. In humans, a comparative, randomized, double-blind study showed that the administration of instant coffee enriched with chlorogenic acid induced a reduction in body fat and body mass at least in part due to a reduction in the absorption of glucose [179]. In addition, inhibition of the activity of glucose-6-phosphatase would limit the release of glucose into the general circulation [180] and, therefore lower insulin levels. This would ultimately lead to an increase in the consumption of fat reserves, due to the reduced availability of glucose as an energy source [179]. Nonetheless, the efficacy of these products in those already regularly exposed to caffeine remains to be demonstrated. Both coffee drinking and obesity tend to co-exist in most developed societies.

Citrus Aurantium

C. aurantium (Citrus Aurantium extract [®], Bitter Orange extract[®]), also known as bitter orange, sour orange, or Seville orange has been used for thousands of years in ancient Chinese medicine. *C. aurantium* contains alkaloids such as *p*-Octopamine and synephrines which exert adrenergic agonist activity [181] and are present in supplements designed to aid weight loss [182].

Due to their adrenergic agonist properties *C. aurantium* alkaloids are used clinically as decongestants, vasopressors during surgical procedures, for acute treatment of priapism and in ophthalmological exams for pupil dilation [183]. In terms of their effects on body weight, synephrines could potentially increase energy expenditure and decrease food intake [184]. In addition, there is some evidence that adrenergic agonists, including *C. aurantium* synephrines, decrease gastric motility [185].

In vitro studies have shown that synephrines promote lipolysis in adipocytes [186] . In rodents, synephrines administration reduces body weight [185, 187], 188] and increases lipoprotein lipase activity [188]. Nevertheless, similarly to other sympathetic agonists, *C. aurantium* fruit extracts seem to have cardiotoxic effects [189].

In humans a few trials have examined the effects of *C. aurantium* synephrines alone, or in combination with other ingredients, on body weight and/or body composition. Overall, these studies reported a loss of 2.4–3.4 kg among participants using SAs, while placebo groups lost 0.94–2.05 kg [183]. Although these results might suggest some beneficial effects from synephrines supplementation, they cannot be considered conclusive at this point because they do not separate the effects of *C. aurantium* or SAs from those of other ingredients, particularly ephedrine. In addition these trials were of short duration and sample sizes were frequently inadequate. Therefore it can be concluded that since the available data on *C. aurantium* weight loss properties are limited, and its toxic effects relevant, it would be difficult to formulate *C. aurantium* related public health recommendations with confidence.

PHYTOCHEMICALS THAT DECREASE BODY WEIGHT THROUGH A COMBINATION OF CENTRAL AND PERIPHERAL MECHANISMS

Ginseng

Ginseng based supplements (Nature's Resource Ginseng®, Pharmanex® Energy Formula, Puritan's Pride®, Korean Ginseng®, Vitamin World®, Puritan's Pride®, and American Ginseng®) are some of the most popular and highly regarded supplements on the market today.

Ginsenosides have been regarded as the principal components responsible for the pharmacological activities of both Panax ginseng (including red ginseng) and American ginseng (*P. quinquefolium*) [190]. Saponins are extracts of the stem, leaves and roots of both Panax ginseng and American ginseng. They contain several active ginsenosides [191]. *In vivo* studies have shown that saponins from *P. quinquefolium* inhibit pancreatic lipase activity [192]. Studies in rodents have shown that the saponin and purified ginsenosides of ginseng have an anti-obesity effect in dietary and genetically obese rodents [163-166]. The majority of reports agree that the main effect of ginsenosides is the inhibition of pancreatic lipase, however there are other suggested mechanisms which may work independently or concurrently, such as increasing EE, improving sensitivity to insulin and changing blood insulin levels [165, 167, 168] and very interestingly, a central effect in the hypothalamus. A study by Etou et al [193] showed that intracerebroventricular infusion of the ginsenoid Rb-1 potently decreased food intake dose-dependently. The analysis of meal patterns revealed that the suppressive effect was due to decreasing meal size. The anorectic effects of central Rb-1 seem to be site-specific since its administration into the VMH reduced food intake, whereas in the lateral hypothalamus it did not alter intake. The specificity of Rb-1 in reducing meal size suggests a particular action on within-meal controls of food consumption [194]. Very recently, it has been demonstrated that the administration of the ginseng saponins protopanaxadiol and protopanaxatriol to dietary-induced obese rats decreased body weight, total food intake, adiposity, serum total cholesterol and leptin to levels equal to or below the normal diet animals [195]. When investigating the mechanisms responsible for these effects the authors found that the animals that received the saponins had lower level of hypothalamic NPY and higher levels of CCK. These results suggest that the anti-obesity actions of saponins target central and peripheral mechanisms. Whilst these potential mechanisms of action are entirely plausible, the efficacy of ginsenosides in weight management is, as far as we are aware, undemonstrated.

Caffeine

Caffeine (Caffeine Pro[®]) is the most widely consumed behaviourally active substance in the world [196]. Almost all caffeine consumed comes from dietary sources (beverages and food), most of it from coffee and tea [196]. The central effects of caffeine at habitually consumed doses are due to its effects on the widely distributed adenosine A1, A2A and A2B receptors [186, 187]. Adenosine is known to modulate the action of neurotransmitters, including dopamine (DA) in the NAc [197, 198] and PFC [199]. Some studies demonstrate that a functional DA/adenosine interaction in the NAc is necessary to induce the reinforcing effects of rewards [200], and that adenosine is involved in sweet taste perception [201, 202].

Experiments performed in rodents have shown that that long-term consumption of caffeine decreases body weight, body fat mass, adipocyte number and palatable food consumption [155, 203-205]. By blocking adenosine receptors, caffeine could blunt the dopaminergic tone in the NAc and thus decrease the perception of the rewarding effects of palatable food ultimately leading to a decrease in consumption of palatable food. In addition, the effect of caffeine on intake of palatable food could also be the consequence of an increased cholinergic transmission in the NAc. Cholinergic transmission is also related to feeding behaviour as it is a signal of satiation [206, 207], and acute and chronic administration of caffeine increase the release of acetylcholine in the NAc [208]. Moreover, caffeine disrupts operant responding in rats trained to press levers for food rewards, however, tolerance develops to this effect [209]. Apart from its effect on adenosine receptors, it is known that caffeine alters serotonergic and noradrenergic neurotransmission [196]. It has been reported that in addition to decreasing fat deposits, caffeine administration to dietary obese mice increases 5-HT content in several brain structures including the hypothalamus, hippocampus and striatum [210]. This is an interesting finding since 5-HT increases correlate with decreases in appetite [211].

Although long-term intervention studies in humans showed no effect of caffeine consumption on body weight [212-215], acute administration in controlled experiments appears to have a small reducing effect on caloric intake [174, 216-218]. Also, reintroduction of caffeine after a period of abstinence in regular coffee consumers was found to reduce daily EI by decreasing the number of meals [219]. Increased caffeine intake has been reported to produce slightly smaller weight gains in men and women when compared to controls [220]. A possible explanation for the lack of a long-term effect of caffeine is the development of a tolerance to its effects [212].

In addition to its central actions, caffeine has also been reported to reduce body weight through a thermogenic action. However, the thermogenic effect of caffeine seems to be more relevant in normal weight individuals [221-223]. Similarly, caffeine-induced lipolysis seems to be more prominent in non obese subjects [224]. It has been suggested that caffeine inhibits the phosphodiesterase-induced degradation of intracellular cyclic AMP (cAMP) [225]. Furthermore, it has been reported that caffeine stimulates substrate cycles like the Cori cycle (conversion of glycogen and glucose to lactate) and the FFA-triglyceride cycle [226-228]. Caffeine administration to humans increases urinary catecholamine excretion, this effect is mainly on A rather than NA excretion, suggesting that it acts primarily via adrenomedullary stimulation and not through peripheral sympathetic discharge [229]. To conclude, caffeine seems to act through central and peripheral mechanisms which would, over the long term, help with achieving weight loss. However, because of the issue of tolerance, the potential benefits of such an approach to weight control in societies of individuals already exposed to high levels of caffeine may be somewhat limited.

Nicotine

Nicotine is an alkaloid naturally occurring in tobacco leaves [230] and is its major addictive component. Among several effects, nicotine reduces appetite and alters feeding patterns typically resulting in reduced body weight [231]. The results of many epidemiologic studies agree on a strong inverse relationship between cigarette smoking and body weight, with smokers weighing significantly less than non-smokers of the same age and sex [232, 233]. In addition, smoking cessation is usually accompanied by hyperphagia and weight gain which is more prominent in women [234-237]. Similarly to caffeine, nicotine exerts its effect through central and metabolic actions.

Peripherally, nicotine could lead to weight loss by both increasing metabolic rate and decreasing metabolic efficiency. Smoking a single cigarette has been shown to induce a 3% rise in EE within 30 minutes [238]. Although studies of nicotine-induced changes in overall metabolic rate are more variable [239, 240], nicotine administration has been shown to alter metabolic processing *in vivo* (humans and animals) and in both hepatocytes and adipocytes [240-242]. *In vitro* studies have shown that nicotine decreases lipolysis by inhibiting lipoprotein lipase activity, decreasing triglyceride uptake and hence lessening net storage in adipose tissue [240]. Activation of nicotinic receptors in both white and brown adipose tissue induces the expression of uncoupling protein 1 (UCP1) [242]. As UCP1 shifts the balance of energy metabolism from the generation of ATP to the generation of heat, this represents a shift in metabolic efficiency compatible with the average lower bodyweight of smokers [235].

Besides its metabolic properties, nicotine also alters intake and appetite by modulating the central pathways that regulate the various aspects of food ingestion. Studies performed in rodents have shown that the reduction in food intake observed after nicotine administration is associated with contemporary changes in hypothalamic neurotransmitters involved in appetite regulation [243, 244] (for an extensive review see [233]) . For instance, acute and chronic exposure to nicotine decreases hypothalamic NPY levels [219, 245]. Chronic administration of nicotine down regulates orexin binding sites [246]. Moreover, nicotine enhances dopaminergic and serotonergic activity in the LH [233, 247] which may promote satiety, and the increased food intake associated with smoking cessation has been hypothesized to be due to a desensitisation of these neurones [248]. Nicotine also increases DA release in reward areas such as the the NAc [249] and the VTA [250]. However, an attempt to confirm an acute anorectic effect of nicotine mediated by DA or by systemic administration of antagonists prior to nicotine has yielded negative results [251].

In humans, numerous clinical and epidemiological studies indicate that body weight and BMI are lower in cigarette smokers than in non-smokers [252-255]. Body leanness is particularly associated with the duration, rather than the intensity of smoking [232]. Studies of feeding behaviour reveal that although in both smokers and non-smokers nicotine does not change hunger sensations [231], its administration decreases meal size, without substantial changes in meal number [256, 257]. The effects of chronic nicotine administration on appetite suppression, decreased food intake, and leanness are not confined to humans [256, 258, 259]. In rodents, chronic nicotine administration has also been found to cause weight loss or decrements in the rate of weight gain [234, 258-264], an effect which has been found by some studies to be due, in part, to decreased food intake [260, 264, 265]. Due to its abuse potential, nicotine preparations are almost exclusively used to delay post cessation weight gain [266-268]. Moreover, given health and addiction issues surrounding smoking, it is unlikely that non-prescription nicotine based weight control products could enter the market without considerable demonstration of efficacy and absence of psychological side effects both during treatment and at cessation.

Khat

Chewing leaves of the khat plant (*Catha edulis*) is a prevalent social custom in the Republic of Yemen and parts of East Africa [269]. The appetite suppressant effects of khat chewing have been reported for several centuries. As cited by Le Bras and Fretillere [270], Naguib Ad-Din, in 1237 prescribed in his "Livre de médicaments composés" the use of khat by warriors and messengers to relieve tiredness and hunger. Several other more recent reports also mention the anorexigenic effects of *C. edulis* [271, 272]. The predominant active ingredients of *C. edulis* are cathinone (1-a-aminopropiophenone) and cathine (D-nor-pseudoephedrine). These compounds share similarities with amphetamine, with up to 90% being absorbed during chewing, predominantly via the oral mucosa [273].

Amphetamine-like compounds affect appetite centrally, by acting in the hypothalamus. Cathinone and cathine need, like amphetamine, recently synthesized brain cathecolamines to be active [274]. In rats, systemic administration of cathinone and cathine decreases food intake [272, 275]. However, as with amphetamine, tolerance to the anorectic effects of these amines develops after 7 days [272]. Apart from direct effects in the hypothalamus, cathinone also delays gastric emptying. In a placebo-controlled study performed in healthy volunteers, khat chewing prolonged gastric emptying significantly when compared to lettuce chewing. This effect is attributed to the enhanced sympathomimetic action of cathinone [276]. This, together with central effects, explains the correlation between cathinone levels and hunger and fullness scores. However, both effects are likely to be secondary to the central sympathomimetic effect and do not appear to be associated with changes in the levels of peripheral peptides such as ghrelin and PYY [269].

Hoodia Gordonii

H. gordonii (commercially available as pills, patches, and liquid: Hoodia pure[®], Hoodia MAX[®], Pure Hoodia[®], RapidSlim SX[®], Hooderma[®], Hoodia-HG57[®]), a member of the large milkweed family, is a desert-originating, succulent, slow growing plant which is widely distributed through the arid areas of South Africa and Namibia [277]. Anecdotal reports and interviews of native and non-native South Africans, reported that the ingestion of Hoodia sap apparently decreased both the feelings and sensations (e.g., 'pangs') of hunger that occurred during long treks in the dry bush [278] The pharmacological properties of the sap of the Hoodia species (including subspecies *H.* or *H. lugardi*), were examined in detail as part of a project carried out by the National Food Research Institute, CSIR, Pretoria, South Africa in 1963 which investigated more than a thousand species of indigenous plants that were used as food [279]. Preliminary experiments that evaluated the thirst quenching properties of Hoodia extracts in mice also found that the extract had an appetite-suppressant activity. This led to further research and the identification of the active compound which is a tri-rhabinoside, 14-OH, 12-tigloyl pregnane steroidal glycoside [280, 281]. Currently, there are more than twenty international patent applications/ registrations on *H. gordonii* relating to the appetite suppressant, anti-diabetic activity and the treatment of gastric acid secretion [279]. However, the available literature offers limited reports on the biological effects of *H. gordonii* and its active compounds [279]. Initial feeding experiments in rats showed that both the crude extract and the pregnane glycoside, administered over an eight day period, decreased food consumption and body mass when compared to animals receiving placebo [281]. This reduction in body weight has been replicated in a second study in rats [282]. Studies performed in diabetic obese Zucker rats showed that the dried extracts of the plant sap exerted anorectic activity and reversal of diabetes which were maintained for the duration of dosing (up to 8 weeks). Interestingly, the decrease in food intake and subsequent weight loss seemed to be independent of the nutrient content of the diet and also occurred in animals that exposed to a highly palatable diet (Phytopharm and Pfizer, unpublished). In addition, Phytopharm, who in 1997 were granted the license for the patent for the active component of the Hoodia "P57" extract, have recently disclosed phase 1 studies in healthy overweight humans where significant reductions in calorie intake and body weight were achieved [283].

To determine whether P57 exerts its effect through a central mechanism, MacLean and Luo [284] administered the compound directly into the brain ventricles and found a 50-60% decrease in food intake over 24 h. The same study found that P57 increased the ATP content in hypothalamic cells. Increased hypothalamic ATP correlates with decreased appetite, while diet restriction produces a decrease in ATP in the hypothalamus. This assertion is supported by the finding that hypothalamic ATP was reduced after four days of moderate food deprivation, and central administration of P57 was able to reverse this effect [284]. This finding suggests that one mechanism of action of P57 is through a central mechanism. However this by no means rules out the possibility that P57 could also act through a peripheral mechanism, for example on vagal afferent nerves on gastric emptying, or on potentially anorectic peripheral hormones, such as CCK [285]. P57 has been in the market for some time. First developed in partnership with Pfizer for a drug application, and then with Unilever as a food ingredient, the product is currently with an industrial partner. This suggests that it has been difficult to successfully develop P57 as a weight controlling product, which brings into question the potential of hoodia for this type of product per se.

Caralluma Fimbriata

Similarly to *H. gordonii*, *C. fimbriata* (Slimaluma®), is also well known as a famine food, an appetite suppressant, a portable food for hunting and a thirst quencher among tribal populations. *C. fimbriata* is an edible succulent cactus that belongs to the family Asclepiadaceae and is cooked as a vegetable, used in preserves like chutneys and pickles, or eaten raw. There are no adverse event reports on the Indian subcontinent over centuries of use [286]. It is widely found in India, Africa, the Canary Islands, Arabia, southern Europe, Ceylon, and Afghanistan [287].

The key ingredients in *C. fimbriata* are pregnane glycosides, flavone glycosides, megastigmane glycosides, bitter principles, saponins and various other flavonoids [288]. The appetite suppressing action of *C. fimbriata* could be mainly attributed to the pregnane glycosides. These compounds seem to have peripheral and central effects. In the adipose tissue, pregnane glycosides exert their effect at least in part by blocking both ATP-citrate lyase, an extra-mitochondrial enzyme involved in the initial steps of *de novo* lipogenesis [289], and malonyl Coenzyme A [290] leading to a reduction in lipogenesis. In the central structures regulating appetite, pregnane glycosides and its related molecules seem to share a similar mechanism of that of *H. gordonii* where they act by amplifying the signaling of the energy sensing function in the basal hypothalamus [284, 291].

A placebo-controlled randomized trial performed in overweight humans showed that administration of *C. fimbriata* extracts over a period of two months lead to a reduction in self-reported measures of appetite, body weight and waist circumference when compared to a control group [291]. Interestingly *C. fimbriata* selectively reduced the intake of refined sugars, sweets, cholesterol and saturated fats, without altering fruit, vegetable or fish intake. This could provide an additional mechanism of reduction in body weight since the consumption of foods such as whole grains, fruit and vegetables has been found to be directly associated with reduction in hunger and increased satiety levels, which could lead to lowered voluntary EI [292].

Coleus Forskohlii

C. forskohlii (ForsLean®) is a plant native to India that belongs to the mint family and has been used traditionally as a herbal medicine to treat various disorders of the cardiovascular, respiratory, GI, and CN systems [293]. Chemically, it is a plant rich in alkaloids, which are considered likely to have influence on the biological systems [294]. One of the main active compounds in C. *forskohlii* is forskolin, a diterpene that acts directly on adenylate cyclase [295]. Adenylate cyclase is an enzyme that activates cyclic adenosine monophosphate (cAMP). In turn cAMP promotes lipolysis, increases the body's basal metabolic rate, and increases utilisation of body fat [296].

A placebo-controlled randomized trial performed in non dieting overweight women showed that although C. *forskohlii* supplementation did not promote weight loss, it helped mitigate weight gain with apparently no clinically significant side effects [297] . These data would suggest further clinical study of C. *forskohlii* may be worthwhile.

PHYTOCHEMICALS THAT INCREASE APPETITE AND BODY WEIGHT

Cannabis Sativa

Although the use of cannabis (*C. sativa*) for medicinal and other purposes dates back at least four thousand years, understanding of its underlying pharmacology dates back only forty years. Rapid progress in this understanding has only been made since the discovery of the receptors that bind to exogenous as well as the recently discovered endogenous cannabinoids. Cannabis contains more than sixty bioactive 'cannabinoid' compounds [298]. Of these, Δ^9-tetrahydrocannabinol (Δ^9-THC) (Marinol®, Dronabinol®, Sativex®) is widely regarded to be primarily responsible for many of the well-known physiological and psychoactive properties of the plant, and has been the focus of many recent pharmacological and therapeutic developments. Unlike the majority of plant derived drugs, Δ^9-THC is an aromatic hydrocarbon rather than an alkaloid [299].

Cannabinoids are known for their rewarding effects and for their ability to stimulate increases in food intake (i.e. the marijuana 'munchies') [48]. It is now reasonable to assume that cannabis hyperphagia is largely attributable to Δ^9-THC actions at brain CB1 cannabinoid receptors, and reflects a biologically significant role of endocannabinoids in appetite processes. However, despite recent advances in cannabinoid pharmacology and the aforementioned promotion of CB1 antagonists in an anti-obesity role, the past decade has seen surprisingly little progress in our understanding of the mechanisms whereby exogenous or endogenous cannabinoids promote eating.

Typically, healthy volunteers (often experienced marijuana users) show substantial increases in caloric intake, most frequently derived from snack foods after acute and chronic dosing (typically in the form of cannabis cigarettes, and less frequently oral Δ^9-THC administration) [48, 300-305]. Δ^9-THC seems to predominantly enhance the orosensory qualities of food, particularly sweet, palatable items [306, 307]. However, it has recently been demonstrated that Δ^9-THC can have broad, dose-related effects on appetite that are not restricted to specific flavours or food types (Townson and Kirkham, unpublished observations). It is probable, but untested, that these actions are CB1 receptor-mediated, since the broader psychological actions of cannabis in people are reversed by the selective CB1 antagonist rimonabant (Acomplia®) [308]. Additionally, a small number of clinical trials have assessed the possible benefits of cannabinoids in the treatment of wasting and appetite loss in cancer cachexia and AIDS. Treatment with Δ^9-THC improved appetite ratings, increased food intake, and attenuated weight loss or induced weight gain [309-312]. In animals, systemic and central administration of Δ^9-THC and endogenous cannabinoids such as anandamide and 2-AG has been shown to stimulate feeding [313-319]. Importantly, this effect has been shown to be mediated by CB1 receptors, being reversed by rimonabant but not the CB2 selective antagonist SR144258 [320]. The hyperphagic effect of Δ^9-THC in rats is also remarkably potent, causing animals to overconsume even when replete. Interestingly, low doses of Δ^8-THC (another phytocannabinoid), have been reported to have significantly greater hyperphagic potency than Δ^9-THC [321]. Such data indicate the importance of exploring the behavioural actions of other phytocannabinoids.

Regarding the relation between reward and appetite effects, a promising hypothesis is that cannabinoids increase appetite and food intake at least in part by enhancing the hedonic impact or palatability of food [322-324]. Systemic and central administration of Δ^9-THC potently increased intake of sweet foods more than less palatable foods [325], and enhanced voluntary licking bouts at a sucrose spout in a manner consistent with palatability enhancement [326]. Moreover, systemic administration of Δ^9-THC in rats is reported to cause eventual increase in affective orofacial 'liking' reactions elicited by the taste of sucrose, suggesting enhancement of taste palatability [323].

The brain substrates of cannabinoid hedonic effects are so far unknown, but hypotheses suggest that endogenous cannabinoid neurotransmission in limbic brain structures such as the NAc mediates the hedonic impact of natural rewards like sweetness [327]. The NAc is an especially likely candidate for cannabinoid mediation of hedonic impact because it is known to contribute to the generation, via other neurotransmitters, of hedonic affect ('liking') and appetitive motivation ('wanting') for food and drug rewards [328].

Sutherlandia (Lessertia Frutescens)

Sutherlandia *(L. frutescens)* is commonly given in the belief that this herb will treat some of the symptoms associated with HIV/AIDS, such as nausea and lack of appetite, amongst others [329]. A recent randomized, double-blind, placebo-controlled trial of *Sutherlandia* leaf powder in healthy adults showed that 800 mg/d during 3 months increased appetite ratings [330]. The constraints of the investigation related to limited sample size, precluding firm conclusions from being drawn about these preliminary data or any speculation related to mechanisms of action.

Chapter 4

CONCLUSION

Overall, no single phytochemical can be considered to a proven weight control product. Whilst, some of the phytochemicals reviewed above show potentially promising effects for weight control, for the majority of cases more data are needed to define safety, the optimal dose required, the mechanism of action and the actual magnitude of effects that can be expected during use in practice. Moreover, many of these substances may also produce substantial and potentially averse side effects.

Moreover, for the majority of compounds described here, there are tantalizing but still inconsistent or incomplete data relating to the mechanism of action and benefits for weight control. In some cases (e.g. *A. turbinata*, sutherlandia), it is not yet even established, even in the most basic terms, what aspects of energy balance (intake, uptake, or expenditure) are actually affected. Some of these phytochemicals probably do not directly affect body weight or weight loss, but could benefit body composition during weight maintenance or (re)gain periods. Other ingredients present significant obstacles to use in foods, because of issues such as safety (caffeine, nicotine, Δ^9-THC, *C. aurantium*). On the other hand, some proposed ingredients (e.g. green tea) could be particularly attractive because they have a long history of safe consumption, and also may bring other added health benefits beyond weight control. For bulk fats such as plant derived oils, the levels that would need to be used may be quite high as a replacement for traditional food oils. This may limit the food formats where they would be of most value, and the putative 'functional' benefit for weight control needs to be balanced against the significant amounts of energy delivered by such ingredients at effective doses.

Additionally, it is important to note here that although some phytochemicals that can be acquired over the counter have been scientifically tested, others have shown no proven efficacy (i.e. *S. matsudana*, caffeine, ginseng).

Improved understanding and evidence on each of the reviewed and other proposed weight control ingredients will guide further research, as well as the selection of ingredients and product formats that can deliver the most attractive and effective benefits to consumers. Ultimately, only randomised, double blinded, placebo-controlled clinical trials of phytochemicals in humans can demonstrate their true potential. With regard to appetite and food intake this will involve proving phytochemical based products significantlu reduce daily caloric intake but adjusting appetite rather than by causing behavioural disruption or inducing malaise. For all ingredient purported to be useful in weight control, significant placebo subtracted weight loss needs be demonstrated at least in the medium term i.e. up to 24 weeks of use.

Table 1. Mechanisms of action of various phytochemicals

Product	Mechanism of action	Ref
Korean pine nut FFA and TG	↑CCK and GLP-1.	[81, 86, 87]
Palm and oat oil (Olibra®)	↑PYY, CCK and GLP-1.	[88]
Gallic acid	Competes with cathecolamines for inactivation via COMT. Inhibits SE and decreases lipid absorption.	[94, 101]
G. cambogia	Inhibits ATP-citrate lyase. Alters the expression of adipogenesis related genes.	[110, 111, 118, 119]
S. matsudana (polyphenol extract)	↑NA induced lipolysis. Inhibits α-amylase activity and palmitic acid absorption.	[125]
Platycodi radix saponins	Inhibit pancreatic lipase. ↓ gastric secretion.	[130-132]
K. scoparia saponins and alcohol extract	Inhibit pancreatic lipase.	[134]
A. turbinata escins	Inhibit pancreatic lipase.	[136, 138]
Oolong tea catechins	Inhibit pancreatic lipase.	[139]
Green tea catechins	Inhibit phospho-ERK1, phospho-ERK2, Cdk2, PPARc2, and C/EBP, GI enzymes, COMT, α-amylase and sucrose.	[149, 151-153, 331, 332]
GCBE and chlorogenic acid	Enhances CPT activity. ↓ Glucose absorption.	[178, 179]
C. aurantium synephrines	Adrenergic agonist activity, ↑ EE and ↓ gut motility.	[183]
Ginseng saponins	Inhibit pancreatic lipase. ↑CCK. ↓ NPY in the hypothalamus.	[192, 195]
Caffeine	CNS: Blocks adenosine receptors, ↓ DA transmission in NAc. ↑ DA in PFC. ↑ cholinergic transmission. Alters 5-HT transmission. Peripheral: ↑ thermogenesis.	[156, 184, 225-229]
Nicotine	CNS: ↑DA release in LHA, NAc and VTA. ↑ 5-HT release. Modulates orexin neurotransmission Peripheral: inhibits lipoprotein lipase. Induces the expression of UCP-1.	[233, 240, 242, 246, 247, 249, 250]
Khat cathinone and cathine	↑ sympathetic activity. Delay gastric emptying.	[272]
Hoodia gordoni extract	↑ ATP content in hypothalamic cells.	[284]

Table 1. (Continued).

Product	Mechanism of action	Ref
C. fimbriata	CNS: ↑ ATP content in hypothalamic cells. Peripheral: Inhibits ATP–citrate lyase and malonyl CoA.	[284, 289-291]
C. forskohlii	Stimulates adenyl cyclase. ↑ cAMP.	[296]
THC	Modulates opioid and DA neurotransmission in CNS rewarding areas.	[322-324]

Table 2. *In vitro* **effects of phytochemicals and their doses**

Product	Dose	Effect	Ref
Korean pine nut FFA	50 μM	↑ CCK-8 release.	[81]
G. cambogia HCA SX	10 μM-1 mM	↑ 5-HT release in isolated rat brain cortex. Lowers abdominal fat leptin expression.	[333, 334]
S. matsudana (polyphenol extract)	250–5000 g/mL	↑ NA induced lypolisis. Inhibits α-amylase activity. Inhibits of palmitic acid absorption.	[125]
K. scoparia alcohol extract and saponins	0.5 and 1.0 g/L	Inhibits pancreatic lipase.	[130, 132]
A. turbinata escins	0.25 mg/ml	Inhibit pancreatic lipase.	[134]
Oolong tea catechins	20-100 μM	Inhibit pancreatic lipase.	[136]
Green tea catechins	05-2 g/L	Inhibit pancreatic lipase.	[139]
	5 -30 μM	Inhibit adipocytes differentiation Inhibit α-amylase and sucrase.	[148-150, 152]
C. aurantium synephrines	0.1 μM	↑ lipolysis	[186]
H. gordonii	5000 nM	↑ ATP content in hypothalamic cells.	[284]

Table 3. *In vivo* effects of Phytochemicals, their routes of administration and doses

Product	Dose	Effect	Ref
Korean pine nut FFA and TG	Humans: 2-3g/day VO	↑ CCK and GLP-1 ↓ Desire to eat and prospective food intake.	[81, 86, 87, 89]
Palm and oat oil (Olibra®)	Humans: 5-15 g/day VO	↓ Food intake. ↓ Hunger and desire to eat.	[88, 92, 93]
Gallic acid	Rats: 360 mg IV, 400 mg intragastric. 1-5% of diet. 2% IP infusion. Humans: 2.4 g/day VO	↓ Food intake. No effect.	[94, 97] [97]
G. cambogia (HCA)	Rodents: 0, 0.2, 2.0 and 5.0% of feed intake, 52.6 mmol OH-CIT/kg in diet. Humans 900, 2800 mg/day VO	↓ EI, body weight, visceral fat, leptin levels and adipocyte size. ↑ EE. ↓ EI and body weight. Sustained satiety.	[109-111, 333, 334] [115, 116]
S. matsudana (polyphenol extract)	Mice: 5% polyphenol fraction in diet	↓ Adiposity and body weight.	[125]
Platycodi radix saponins	Dietary obese rodents: 35- 70 mg / kg VO	↓ Body weight and caloric intake.	[130, 132]
K. scoparia	Rodents: 1-3% in diet	↓ Body weight increase induced by high fat diet.	[134]
A. turbinata escins	Dietary obese mice: 1 mg/kg VO Mice: 100 mg/kg VO	↓ Body weight increase -induced by high fat diet. Attenuates increase in glucose levels.	[136, 138]

Table 3. (Continued).

Product	Dose	Effect	Ref
Oolong tea catechins	Rodents: 0.5% in diet. 690 mg of catechins	↓ Body weight increase -induced by high fat diet. ↓ Adipocyte size ↓ body weight, BMI and adiposity.	[139, 142]
Green tea catechins	Rats: 20 gr/kg in drinking water. EGCG: 75-85 mg/kg i.p. Humans: 130-600 mg/day alone or in combination with caffeine.	↓ Adiposity. ↓ Body weight and adiposity.	[160-164, 335, 336]
Green coffee bean extract (GCBE) and chlorogenic acid	Mice: GCBE (0.5-1% in diet or 200-400 mg/kg VO), Chlorogenic acid: (0.15-0.3% in diet or 60-120mg/kg VO) Humans: 140 mg/d VO	↓ Body weight and visceral fat. ↓ Hepatic TG levels. ↓ Glucose absorption. ↓ BMI and adiposity.	[178, 179]
C. aurantium synephrine	Rodents: 10mg/kg IP Humans: 32-300 mg/d VO	↓ Lipoprotein lipase activity. ↓ Body weight	[187, 188, 337]
Ginseng saponins	Rodents: 1-3% of diet, 50-250mg/kg IP 0.05, 0.10 and 0.20 µ mol ICV	↓ Food intake, body weight and adiposity.	[192, 193, 195, 338]
Caffeine	Rats: 1g/L drinking water Humans: 50-100 mg VO	↓ Palatable food intake, ↓ adiposity. Slight anorectic effect.	[205, 210]

Product	Dose	Effect	Ref
Nicotine	Rats: µM in LHA, NAc by microdialysis. 0.5-12 mg/kg SC or IP Humans: smoking chewing gum and patches	↓ Food intake and body weight	[231, 240, 247, 249, 262, 339, 340]
Khat cathinone and cathine	Rats: 4-10 mg/kg rats IP	↓ Food intake and body weight. ↓ Food intake	[272, 275]
H. gordonii extract	Rats: 0.4–40 nmol ICV Humans: 500-750 mg/day VO	↓ Food intake and body weight. ↓ Food intake and body weight	[284]
C. fimbriata extract	Humans 1 g/day VO	↓ Hunger levels, food intake, body weight and waist circumference	[291]
C. forskohlii	Overweight women: 250 mg/day VO	Prevents weight gain	[297]
Δ⁹-THC	Rodents: 0.5-4 mg/kg VO, SC, IP. 2.5, 10 and 25 µg ICV Humans: smoking cigarettes with 1.8-3.1% THC, 20-210 mg/day VO	↑ Food intake and body weight ↑ Food intake and body weight	[48, 300-305, 314, 315, 317, 319-321, 341, 342]
Sutherlandia	800 mg/d for 3 months	↑ Appetite ratings	[330]

Table 4. Effects on food intake and / or body weight of various phytochemicals and their recommended uses

Product	Acute effect	Chronic effect	Recommended use	Ref
Korean pine nut	↓ 9% ad libitum food intake		Supports long term weight loss.	[87]
Palm and oat oil (Olibra®)	↓ Energy (25%) and macronutrient intake up to 36 h post-consumption	Helps to maintain weight after weight loss programmes.	Helps weight maintenance after weight loss programmes.	[89]
Gallic acid		No dose-related weight loss or reduction in food intake.	Not conclusive	[97]
G. cambogia (HCA)		5.4% and 5.2% in baseline body weight and BMI. ↓ 24 h EI by 15-30%	Helps weight maintenance after weight loss programmes.	[115, 116]
S. matsudana			No human studies.	
Platycodi radix			No human studies.	
K. scoparia turbinata			No human studies.	
Oolong tea saponins		↓ body weight (1.5%), BMI (1.5%), waist circumference (2.0%), body fat mass (3.7%)	As an adjuvant in weight loss programmes.	[142]
Green tea		↓ body weight 0.6 –1.25 kg, ↓ body fat 0.5–1.8 kg	As an adjuvant in the management of obesity.	[163-167]
CGBE (chlorogenic acid)		↓ 5.7 kg when compared to placebo	As an adjuvant in the management of obesity.	[179]
C. aurantium synephrine	↑ Heart rate and blood pressure	↓.4–3.4 kg compared to 0.94–2.05 kg in placebo	Use limited by side effects.	[185, 189]
Ginseng saponins			No human studies	

Product	Acute effect	Chronic effect	Recommended use	Ref
Caffeine	↓ 3% EI compared to placebo	No effect	Not conclusive	[174, 213, 343]
Nicotine		Less weight gain (0.47 kg vs 1.02 kg) in smoking cessation programmes	Delay post cessation weight gain.	[268]
Khat			No human studies.	
H. gordonii		↓ EI to 1000 kcal/d	Not conclusive.	[279, 283]
fimbriata		↓ Hunger levels. Non significant trend towards ↓EI, BMI and body weight.	Helps to suppress appetite during weight loss programmes.	[291]
forskohlii			No human studies	
Δ⁹-THC	↑ Appetite, enhances hedonic qualities of food	Attenuates weight loss or induces weight gain	Could helps in the management of appetite and weight in cachexia/cancer/AIDS.	[309-312]
Sutherlandia		↑ appetite ratings	Could help in the management of appetite and weight in cachexia/cancer/AIDS.	[330]

REFERENCES

[1]   Prentice, AM. Early influences on human energy regulation: thrifty genotypes and thrifty phenotypes. *Physiol. Behav*, 2005 86: 640-645.

[2]   Berthoud, HR; Morrison, C. The brain, appetite, and obesity. *Annu. Rev. Psychol*, 2008 59: 55-92.

[3]   Bray, GA. Medical consequences of obesity. *J. Clin. Endocrinol. Metab*, 2004 89: 2583-2589.

[4]   Wadden, TA. Treatment of obesity by moderate and severe caloric restriction. Results of clinical research trials. *Ann. Intern. Med*, 1993 119: 688-693.

[5]   Rosenbaum, M; Leibel, RL. The physiology of body weight regulation: relevance to the etiology of obesity in children. *Pediatrics*, 1998 101: 525-539.

[6]   Dulloo, AG; Jacquet, J; Girardier, L. Poststarvation hyperphagia and body fat overshooting in humans: a role for feedback signals from lean and fat tissues. *Am. J. Clin. Nutr*, 1997 65: 717-723.

[7]   Dulloo, AG; Jacquet, J. Adaptive reduction in basal metabolic rate in response to food deprivation in humans: a role for feedback signals from fat stores. *Am. J. Clin. Nutr*, 1998 68: 599-606.

[8]   Silverstone, T. Appetite suppressants: a review. *Drugs*, 1992 43: 820-836.

[9]   Khan, MA; Herzog, CA; St. Peter, JV; Hartley, GG; Madlon-Kay, R; Dick, CD; Asinger, RW; Vessey, JT. The prevalence of cardiac valvular insufficiency assessed by transthoracic echocardiography in obese patients treated with appetite-suppressant drugs. *N. Engl. J. Med*, 1998 339: 713-718.

[10] Dogangun, B; Bolat, N; Rustamov, I; Kayaalp, L. Sibutramine-induced psychotic episode in an adolescent. *J Psychosom Res*, 2008 65: 505-506.

[11] Taflinski, T; Chojnacka, J. Sibutramine-associated psychotic episode. *Am. J. Psychiatry*, 2000 157: 2057-2058.

[12] Benazzi, F. Organic hypomania secondary to sibutramine-citalopram interaction. *J. Clin. Psychiatry*, 2002 63: 165.

[13] Binkley, K; Knowles, SR. Sibutramine and panic attacks. *Am. J. Psychiatry*, 2002 159: 1793-1794.

[14] Lee, J; Teoh, T; Lee, TS. Catatonia and psychosis associated with sibutramine: a case report and pathophysiologic correlation. *J. Psychosom. Res*, 2008 64: 107-109.

[15] King, DJ; Devaney, N. Clinical pharmacology of sibutramine hydrochloride (BTS 54 524), a new antidepressant, in healthy volunteers. *Br. J. Pharmacol*, 1988 26: 607-611.

[16] Weintraub, M; Rubio, A; Golik, A; Byrne, L; Scheinbaum, ML. Sibutramine in weight control: a dose-ranging, efficacy study. *Clin. Pharmacol. Ther*, 1991 50: 330-337.

[17] Sharma, AM; Caterson, ID; Coutinho, W; Finer, N; Van Gaal, L; Maggioni, AP; Torp-Pedersen, C; Bacher, HP; Shepherd, GM; James, WP. Blood pressure changes associated with sibutramine and weight management - an analysis from the 6-week lead-in period of the sibutramine cardiovascular outcomes trial (SCOUT). *Diabetes Obes. Metab*, 2008.

[18] Maggioni, AP; Caterson, I; Coutinho, W; Finer, N; Gaal, LV; Sharma, AM; Torp-Pedersen, C; Bacher, P; Shepherd, G; Sun, R; James, P. Tolerability of sibutramine during a 6-week treatment period in high-risk patients with cardiovascular disease and/or diabetes: a preliminary analysis of the Sibutramine Cardiovascular Outcomes (SCOUT) Trial. *J. Cardiovasc. Pharmacol*, 2008 52: 393-402.

[19] Cummings, S; Parham, ES; Strain, GW. Position of the American Dietetic Association: Weight management. *J. Am. Diet. Assoc*, 2002 102: 1145-1155.

[20] Halford, JCG. Pharmacotherapy for obesity. *Appetite*, 2006: 6-10.

[21] Filippatos, TD; Derdemezis, CS; Gazi, IF; Nakou, ES; Mikhailidis, DP; Elisaf, MS. Orlistat-associated adverse effects and drug interactions: a critical review. *Drug Saf*, 2008 31: 53-65.

[22] Jequier, E; Tappy, L. Regulation of body weight in humans. *Physiol. Rev*, 1999 79: 451-480.

[23] Zhang, Y; Proenca, R; Maffei, M; Barone, M; Leopold, L; Friedman, JM. Positional cloning of the mouse obese gene and its human homologue. *Nature*, 1994 372: 425-432.

[24] Schwartz, M; Peskind, E; Raskind, M; Boyko, E; Porte, DJ. Cerebrospinal fluid leptin levels: relationship to plasma levels and to adiposity in humans. *Nat. Med*, 1996 2: 589-593.

[25] Woods, S; Seeley, C; Porte, RJJ; Schwartz, M. Signals that regulate food intake and energy homeostasis. *Science*, 1998 280: 1478-1383.

[26] Bagdade, JD; Bierman, E; Porte, D. The significance of basal insulin levels in the evaluation of the insulin response to glucose in diabetic and nondiabetic subjects. *J. Clin. Invest*, 1967 46: 1549-1557.

[27] Reinehr, T; Roth, C; Menke, T; Andler, W. Adiponectin before and after weight loss in obese children. *J. Clin. Endocrinol. Metab*, 2004 89: 3790-3794.

[28] Kojima, M; Hosoda, H; Date, Y; Nakazato, M; Matsuo, H; Kangawa, K. Ghrelin is a growth-hormone-releasing acylated peptide from stomach. *Nature*, 1999 402: 656-660.

[29] Wynne, K; Stanley, S; McGowan, B; Bloom, S. Appetite control. *J. Endocrinol*, 2005 184: 291-318.

[30] Morton, GJ; Cummings, DE; Baskin, DG; Barsh, GS; Schwartz, MW. Central nervous system control of food intake and body weight. *Nature*, 2006 443: 289-295.

[31] Gibbs, J; Young, RC; Smith, GP. Cholecystokinin decreases food intake in rats. *J. Comp. Physiol. Psychol*, 1973 84: 488-495.

[32] Kissileff, HR; Pi-Sunyer, FX; Thornton, J; Smith, GP. C-terminal octapeptide of cholecystokinin decreases food intake in man. *Am. J. Clin. Nutr*, 1981 34: 154-160.

[33] Lieverse, RJ; Jansen, JBMJ; Masclee, AAM; Lamers, CBHW. Role of cholecystokinin in the regulation of satiation and satiety in humans. *Ann. N.Y. Acad. Sci*, 1994 713: 268-272.

[34] Kalra, S; Dube, M; Pu, S; Xu, B; TL, H; Kalra , P. Interacting appetite-regulating pathways in the hypothalamic regulation of body weight. *Endocr. Rev*, 1999 20: 68-100.

[35] Cowley, MA; Smart, JL; Rubinstein, M; Cerdan, MG; Diano, S; Horvath, TL; Cone, RD; Low, MJ. Leptin activates anorexigenic POMC neurons through a neural network in the arcuate nucleus. *Nature*, 2001 411: 480-484.

[36] Elmquist, JK; Elias, CF; Saper, CB. From lesions to leptin: hypothalamic control of food intake and body weight. *Neuron*, 1999 22: 221-232.

[37] Spanswick, D; Smith, MA; Mirshamsi, S; Routh, VH; Ashford, ML. Insulin activates ATP-sensitive K+ channels in hypothalamic neurons of lean, but not obese rats. *Nat. Neurosci*, 2000 3: 757-758.

[38] Elias, CF; Saper, CB; Maratos-Flier, E; Tritos, NA; Lee, C; Kelly, J; Tatro, JB; Hoffman, GE; Ollmann, MM; Barsh, GS; Sakurai, T; Yanagisawa, M; Elmquist, JK. Chemically defined projections linking the mediobasal hypothalamus and the lateral hypothalamic area. *J. Comp. Neurol*, 1998 402: 442-459.

[39] Elias, CF; Aschkenasi, C; Lee, C; Kelly, J; Ahima, RS; Bjorbaek, C; Flier, JS; Saper, CB; Elmquist, JK. Leptin differentially regulates NPY and POMC neurons projecting to the lateral hypothalamic area. *Neuron*, 1999 23: 775-786.

[40] Valassi, E; Scacchi, M; Cavagnini, F. Neuroendocrine control of food intake. *Nutr. Metab. Cardiovasc. Dis*, 2008 18: 158-168.

[41] Sakurai, T; Amemiya, A; Ishii, M; Matsuzaki, I; Chemelli, R; Tanaka, H; Williams, S; Richarson, J; Kozlowski, G; Wilson, S; Arch, J; Buckingham, R; Haynes, A; Carr, S; Annan, R; McNulty, D; Liu, W; Terrett, J; Elshourbagy, N; Bergsma, D; Yanagisawa, M. Orexins and orexin receptors: a family of hypothalamic neuropeptides and G protein-coupled receptors that regulate feeding behavior. *Cell*, 1998 92: 573-585.

[42] Qu, D; Ludwig, DS; Gammeltoft, S; Piper, M; Pelleymounter, MA; Cullen, MJ; Mathes, WF; Przypek, R; Kanarek, R; Maratos-Flier, E. A role for melanin-concentrating hormone in the central regulation of feeding behaviour. *Nature*, 1996 380: 243-247.

[43] Abizaid, A; Gao, Q; Horvath, TL. Thoughts for food: brain mechanisms and peripheral energy balance. *Neuron*, 2006 51: 691-702.

[44] Breivogel, CS; Childers, SR. The functional neuroanatomy of brain cannabinoid receptors. *Neurobiol. Dis*, 1998 5: 417-431.

[45] Fride, E; Ginzburg, Y; Breuer, A; Bisogno, T; Di Marzo, V; Mechoulam, R. Critical role of the endogenous cannabinoid system in mouse pup suckling and growth. *Eur. J. Pharmacol*, 2001 419: 207-214.

[46] De Petrocellis, L; Melck, D; Bisogno, T; Milone, A; Di Marzo, V. Finding of the endocannabinoid signalling system in Hydra, a very primitive organism: possible role in the feeding response. *Neuroscience*, 1999 92: 377-387.

[47] Kirkham, TC; Williams, CM; Fezza, F; Di Marzo, V. Endocannabinoid levels in rat limbic forebrain and hypothalamus in relation to fasting, feeding and satiation: stimulation of eating by 2-arachidonoyl glycerol. *Br. J. Pharmacol*, 2002 136: 550-557.

[48] Greenberg, I; Kuehnle, J; Mendelson, JH; Bernstein, JG. Effects of marihuana use on body weight and caloric intake in humans. *Psychopharmacology (Berl)*, 1976 49: 79-84.

[49] Abel, EL. Cannabis: effects on hunger and thirst. *Behavioral Biology*, 1975 15: 255-281.

[50] Colombo, G; Agabio, R; Diaz, G; Lobina, C; Reali, R; Gessa, GL. Appetite suppression and weight loss after the cannabinoid antagonist SR 141716. *Life Sci*, 1998 63: PL113-7.

[51] Friedman, JM; Halaas, JL. Leptin and the regulation of body weight in mammals. *Nature*, 1998 395: 763-770.

[52] Di Marzo, V; Goparaju, SK; Wang, L; Liu, J; Batkai, S; Jarai, Z; Fezza, F; Miura, G; Palmiter, RD; Sugiura, T; Kunos, G. Leptin-regulated endocannabinoids are involved in maintaining food intake. *Nature*, 2001 410: 822-825.

[53] Bittencourt, JC; Elias, CF. Melanin-concentrating hormone and neuropeptide EI projections from the lateral hypothalamic area and zona incerta to the medial septal nucleus and spinal cord: a study using multiple neuronal tracers. *Brain Res*, 1998 805: 1-19.

[54] Broberger, C; De Lecea, L; Sutcliffe, JG; Hokfelt, T. Hypocretin/orexin- and melanin-concentrating hormone-expressing cells form distinct populations in the rodent lateral hypothalamus: relationship to the neuropeptide Y and agouti gene-related protein systems. *J. Comp. Neurol*, 1998 402: 460-474.

[55] Peyron, C; Tighe, DK; van den Pol, AN; de Lecea, L; Heller, HC; Sutcliffe, JG; Kilduff, TS. Neurons containing hypocretin (orexin) project to multiple neuronal systems. *J. Neurosci*, 1998 18: 9996-10015.

[56] Stratford, T; Kelley, A. Evidence of a functional relationship between the nucleus accumbens shell and lateral hypothalamus subserving the control of feeding behavior. *J. Neurosci*, 1999 19: 11040-11048.

[57] Pajolla, GP; Crippa, GE; Correa, SA; Moreira, KB; Tavares, RF; Correa, FM. The lateral hypothalamus is involved in the pathway mediating the hypotensive response to cingulate cortex-cholinergic stimulation. *Cell Mol. Neurobiol*, 2001 21: 341-356.

[58] Fadel, J; Deutch, AY. Anatomical substrates of orexindopamine interactions: lateral hypothalamic projections to the ventral tegmental area. *Neuroscience*, 2002 111: 379-387.

[59] Berthoud, HR. Multiple neural systems controlling food intake and body weight. *Neurosci. Biobehav. Rev*, 2002 26: 393-428.

[60] Broberger, C. Brain regulation of food intake and appetite: molecules and networks. *J. Intern. Med*, 2005 258: 301-327.

[61] Danforth, EJ; Burger, A. The role of thyroid hormones in the control of energy expenditure. *Clin. Endocrinol. Metab*, 1984 13: 581-595.

[62] Silva, JE. The multiple contributions of thyroid hormone to heat production. *J. Clin. Invest*, 2001 108: 35-37.

[63] Paddon-Jones, D; Westman, E; Mattes, RD; Wolfe, RR; Astrup, A; Westerterp-Plantenga, M. Protein, weight management, and satiety. *Am. J. Clin. Nutr*, 2008 87: 1558S-1561S.

[64] Kim, B. Thyroid hormone as a determinant of energy expenditure and the basal metabolic rate. *Thyroid*, 2008 18: 141-144.

[65] Morrison, SF; Nakamura, K; Madden, CJ. Central control of thermogenesis in mammals. *Exp. Physiol*, 2008 93: 773-797.

[66] Tappy, L. Thermic effect of food and sympathetic nervous system activity in humans. *Reprod. Nutr. Dev*, 1996 36: 391-397.

[67] van Baak, MA. Meal-induced activation of the sympathetic nervous system and its cardiovascular and thermogenic effects in man. *Physiol. Behav*, 2008 94: 178-186.

[68] Welle, S; Lilavivat, U; Campbell, RG. Thermic effect of feeding in man: increased plasma norepinephrine levels following glucose but not protein or fat consumption. *Metabolism*, 1981 30: 953-958.

[69] van Baak, MA. The peripheral sympathetic nervous system in human obesity. *Obes. Rev*, 2001 2: 3-14.

[70] Blaak, EE; van Baak, MA; Kester, AD; Saris, WH. Beta-adrenergically mediated thermogenic and heart rate responses: effect of obesity and weight loss. *Metabolism*, 1995 44: 520-524.

[71] Seals, DR; Bell, C. Chronic sympathetic activation: consequence and cause of age-associated obesity? *Diabetes*, 2004 53: 276-284.

[72] Rosenbaum, M; Hirsch, J; Gallagher, DA; Leibel, RL. Long-term persistence of adaptive thermogenesis in subjects who have maintained a reduced body weight. *Am. J. Clin. Nutr*, 2008 88: 906-912.

[73] Jebb, SA. Metabolic response to slimming, In: Cottrell, R, editor. *Weight Control: The Current Perspective*. London: Chapman & Hall; 1995.

[74] Ravussin, E; Schutz, Y; Acheson, KJ; Dusmet, M; Bourquin, L; Jequier, E. Short-term, mixed-diet overfeeding in man: no evidence for "luxuskonsumption". *Am. J. Physiol*, 1985 249: E470-477.

[75] Salas-Salvado, J; Fernandez-Ballart, J; Ros, E; Martinez-Gonzalez, MA; Fito, M; Estruch, R; Corella, D; Fiol, M; Gomez-Gracia, E; Aros, F; Flores, G; Lapetra, J; Lamuela-Raventos, R; Ruiz-Gutierrez, V; Bullo, M; Basora, J; Covas, MI. Effect of a Mediterranean diet supplemented with nuts on metabolic syndrome status: one-year results of the PREDIMED randomized trial. *Arch. Intern. Med*, 2008 168: 2449-2458.

[76] Fraser, GE; Sabate, J; Beeson, WL; Strahan, TM. A possible protective effect of nut consumption on risk of coronary heart disease. *The Adventist Health Study Arch. Intern. Med*, 1992 1524: 1416-1424.

[77] Hu, FB; Stampfer, MJ; Manson, JE; Rimm, EB; Colditz, GA; Rosner, BA; Speizer, FE; Hennekens, CH; Willett, WC. Frequent nut consumption and risk of coronary heart disease in women: prospective cohort study. *BMJ*, 1998 317: 1341-1345.

[78] Alper, CM; Mattes, RD. Effects of chronic peanut consumption on energy balance and hedonics. *Int. J. Obes. Relat. Metab. Disord*, 2000 26: 1129-1137.

[79] Lee, JW; Lee, KW; Lee, SW; Kim, IH; Rhee, C. Selective increase in pinolenic acid (all-cis-5,9,12-18:3) in Korean pine nut oil by crystallization and its effect on LDL-receptor activity. *Lipids*, 2004 39: 383-387.

[80] Asset, G; Staels, B; Wolff, RL; Baugé, E; Madj, Z; Fruchart, JC; Dallongeville, J. Effects of Pinus pinaster and Pinus koraiensis seed oil supplementation on lipoprotein metabolism in the rat. *Lipids*, 1999 34: 39-44.

[81] Pasman, WJ; Heimerikx, J; Rubingh, CM; van den Berg, R; O'Shea, M; Gambelli, L; Hendriks, HF; Einerhand, AW; Scott, C; Keizer, HG; Mennen, LI. The effect of Korean pine nut oil on in vitro CCK release, on appetite sensations and on gut hormones in post-menopausal overweight women. *Lipids Health Dis*, 2008 7: 10.

[82] Matzinger, D; Degen, L; Drewe, J; Meuli, J; Duebendorfer, R; Ruckstuhl, N; D'Amato, M; Rovati, L; Beglinger, C. The role of long chain fatty acids in regulating food intake and cholecystokinin release in humans. *Gut*, 2000 46: 688-693.

[83] Feltrin, KL; Little, TJ; Meyer, JH; Horowitz, M; Smout, AJ; Wishart, J; Pilichiewicz, AN; Rades, T; Chapman, IM; Feinle-Bisset, C. Effects of intraduodenal fatty acids on appetite, antropyloroduodenal motility, and

plasma CCK and GLP-1 in humans vary with their chain length. *Am. J. Physiol. Regul. Integr. Comp. Physiol*, 2004 287: R524-R533.

[84] McLaughlin, J; Grazia Luca, M; Jones, MN; D'Amato, M; Dockray, G; Thompson, DG. Fatty acid chain length determines cholecystokinin secretion and effect on human gastric motility. *Gastroenterology* 1999 116: 46-53.

[85] Lawton, CL; Delargy, HJ; Brockman, J; Smith, FC; E, BJ. The degree of saturation of fatty acids influences post-ingestive satiety. *Br. J. Nutr*, 2000 83: 473-482.

[86] Scott, C; Pasman, W; Hiemerikx, J; Rubingh, C; Van Den Berg, R; O'Shea, M; Gambelli, L; Hendricks, H; Mennen, L; Einerhand, A. Pinnothin™ suppresses appetite in overweight women. *Appetite*, 2007 49: 330.

[87] Hughes, GM; Boyland, EJ; Williams, NJ; Mennen, L; Scott, C; Kirkham, TC; Harrold, JA; Keizer, HG; Halford, JC. The effect of Korean pine nut oil (PinnoThin) on food intake, feeding behaviour and appetite: a double-blind placebo-controlled trial. *Lipids Health Dis*, 2008 7: 6.

[88] Burns, AA; Livingstone, MB; Welch, RW; Dunne, A; Rowland, IR. Dose-response effects of a novel fat emulsion (Olibra) on energy and macronutrient intakes up to 36 h post-consumption. *Eur. J. Clin. Nutr*, 2002 56: 368-377.

[89] Diepvens, K; Soenen, S; Steijns, J; Arnold, M; Westerterp-Plantenga, M. Long-term effects of consumption of a novel fat emulsion in relation to body-weight management. *Int. J. Obes. (Lond)*, 2007 31: 942-949.

[90] Welch, I; Saunders, K; Read, NW. Effect of ileal and intravenous infusions of fat emulsions on feeding and satiety in human volunteers. *Gastroenterology*, 1985 89: 1293-1297.

[91] Welch, IM; Sepple, CP; Read, NW. Comparisons of the effects on satiety and eating behaviour of infusion of lipid into the different regions of the small intestine. *Gut*, 1988 29: 306-311.

[92] Burns, AA; Livingstone, MB; Welch, RW; Dunne, A; Robson, PJ; Lindmark, L; Reid, CA; Mullaney, U; Rowland, IR. Short-term effects of yoghurt containing a novel fat emulsion on energy and macronutrient intakes in non-obese subjects. *Int. J. Obes. Relat. Metab. Disord*, 2000 24: 1419-1425.

[93] Diepvens, K; Steijns, J; Zuurendonk, P; Westerterp-Plantenga, MS. Short-term effects of a novel fat emulsion on appetite and food intake. *Physiol. Behav*, 2008 95: 114-117.

[94] Glick, Z. Modes of action of gallic acid in suppressing food intake of rats. *J. Nutr*, 1981 111: 1910-1916.

[95] Joslyn, MA; Glick, Z. Comparative effects of gallotannic acid and related phenolics on the growth of rats. *J. Nutr*, 1969 98: 119-126.

[96] Mueller, WS. The significance of tannic substances and theobromine in chocolate milk. *J. Dairy Sci*, 1942 25: 221-230.

[97] Roberts, AT; Martin, CK; Liu, Z; Amen, RJ; Woltering, EA; Rood, JC; Caruso, MK; Yu, Y; Xie, H; Greenway, FL. The safety and efficacy of a dietary herbal supplement and gallic acid for weight loss. *J. Med. Food*, 2007 10: 184-188.

[98] Axelrod, J; Senoh, S; Witkop, B. O-methylation of catecholamines in vivo. *J. Biol. Chem*, 1958 233: 697-701.

[99] Russek, M; Mogenson, G; Stevenson, JA. Calorigenic hyperglycemia and anorexigenic effects of adrenaline and noradrenaline. *Physiol. Behavior*, 1967 2: 429-433.

[100] Abe, I; Prestwich, GD. *Comprehensive Natural Products Chemistry*. Oxford, Pergamon; 1999.

[101] Jang, A; Srinivasan, P; Lee, NY; Song, HP; Lee, JW; Lee, M; Jo, C. Comparison of hypolipidemic activity of synthetic gallic acid-linoleic acid ester with mixture of gallic acid and linoleic acid, gallic acid, and linoleic acid on high-fat diet induced obesity in C57BL/6 Cr Slc mice. *Chem. Biol. Interact*, 2008 174: 109-117.

[102] Lewis, YS; Neelakantan, S. (−)-Hydroxycitric acid - the principal acid in the fruits of Garcinia cambogia. *Desr. Psytochem*, 1965 4: 619-625.

[103] Clouatre, D; Rosenbaum, ME. *The Diet and Health Benefits of HCA*. New Canaan, Connecticut, Keats Publishing; 1994.

[104] Sergio, W. A natural food, the Malabar Tamarind, may be effective in the treatment of obesity. *Med. Hypotheses*, 1988 27: 39-40.

[105] Heymsfield, SB; Allison, D; Vasselli, JR; Pietrobelli, A; Greenfield, D; Nuñez, C. Garcinia cambogia (hydroxycitric acid) as a potential antiobesity agent: a randomized controlled trial. *JAMA*, 1998 280: 1596-1600.

[106] Sullivan, AC; Hamilton, JG; Miller, ON; Wheatley, VR. Inhibition of lipogenesis in rat liver by (−)-hydroxycitrate. *Arch. Biochem. Biophys*, 1972 150: 183-190.

[107] Sullivan, AC; Triscari, J; Hamilton, JG; Miller, ON. Effect of (-)-hydroxycitrate upon the accumulation of lipid in the rat. II. appetite. *Lipids*, 1974 9: 129-134.

[108] Sullivan, AC; Triscari, J; Hamilton, JG; Miller, ON; Wheatley, VR. Effect of (-)-hydroxycitrate upon the accumulation of lipid in the rat. I. lipogenesis. *Lipids*, 1974 9: 121-128.

[109] Rao, RN; Sakaria, KK. Lipid-lowering and antiobesity effect of (−)-hydroxycitric acid. *Nutr. Res*, 1988 8: 209-212.

[110] Vasselli, JR; Shane, E; Boozer, CN; Heymsfield, SB. Garcinia cambogia extract inhibits body weight gain via increased Energy Expenditure (EE) in rats. *FASEB J*, 1998 12: A505.

[111] Kim, KY; Lee, HN; Kim, YJ; Park, T. Garcinia cambogia extract ameliorates visceral adiposity in C57BL/6J mice fed on a high-fat diet. *Biosci. Biotechnol. Biochem*, 2008 72: 1772-1780.

[112] Asghar, M; Monjok, E; Kouamou, G; Ohia, SE; Bagchi, D; Lokhandwala, MF. Super CitriMax (HCA-SX) attenuates increases in oxidative stress, inflammation, insulin resistance, and body weight in developing obese Zucker rats. *Mol. Cell Biochem*, 2007 304: 93-99.

[113] Saito, M; Ueno, M; Ogino, S; Kubo, K; Nagata, J; Takeuchi, M. High dose of Garcinia cambogia is effective in suppressing fat accumulation in developing male Zucker obese rats, but highly toxic to the testis. *Food Chem. Toxicol*, 2005 43: 411-419.

[114] Mattes, RD; Bormann, L. Effects of (-)-hydroxycitric acid on appetitive variables. *Physiol. Behav*, 2000 71: 87-94.

[115] Westerterp-Plantenga, MS; Kovacs, EM. The effect of (-)-hydroxycitrate on energy intake and satiety in overweight humans. *Int. J. Obes. Relat. Metab. Disord*, 2002 26: 870-872.

[116] Preuss, HG; Rao, CV; Garis, R; Bramble, J; Ohia, SE; Bagchi, M; Bagchi, D. An overview of the safety and efficacy of a novel, natural(-)-hydroxycitric acid extract (HCA-SX) for weight management. *J. Med*, 2004 35: 33-48.

[117] McCarty, M; Majeed, M. The pharmacology of Citrin, In: Majeed, M, et al., editor. *Citrin®. A revolutionary, herbal approach to weight management*. Burlingame, CA: New Editions Publishing; 1994;p. 34-52.

[118] Sullivan, AC; Singh, M; Srere, PA; Glusker, JP. Reactivity and inhibitor potential of hydroxycitrate isomers with citrate synthase, citrate lyase, and ATP citrate lyase. *J. Biol. Chem*, 1977 252: 7583-7590.

[119] Watson, JA; Fang, M; Lowenstein, JM. Tricarballylate and hydroxycitrate: substrate and inhibitor of ATP: citrate oxaloacetate lyase. *Arch. Biochem. Biophys*, 1969 135: 209-217.

[120] Baird, I; Parsons, R; Howard, AN. Clinical and metabolic studies of chemically defined diets in the management of obesity. *Metabolism*, 1974 23: 654-657.

[121] Silverston, J; Stark, JE; Buckle, R. Hunger during total starvation. *Lancet*, 1966 1: 343-344.

[122] Greenwood, MR; Cleary, MP; Gruen, R; Blase, D; Stern, JS; Triscari, J; Sullivan, AC. Effect of (-)-hydroxycitrate on development of obesity in the Zucker obese rat. *Am. J. Physiol*, 1981 240: E72-E78.

[123] Korenkov, M; Sauerland, S; Junginger, T. Surgery for obesity. *Curr. Opin. Gastroenterol*, 2005 21: 679-683.

[124] Chiasson, JL; Josse, RG; Gomis, R; Hanefeld, M; Karasik, A; Laakso, M. Acarbose for prevention of type 2 diabetes mellitus: the STOP-NIDDM randomised trial. *Lancet*, 2002 359: 2072-2077.

[125] Han, LK; Sumiyoshi, M; Zhang, J; Liu, MX; Zhang, XF; Zheng, YN; Okuda, H; Kimura, Y. Anti-obesity action of Salix matsudana leaves (Part 1). Anti-obesity action by polyphenols of Salix matsudana in high fat-diet treated rodent animals. *Phytother. Res*, 2003 17: 1188-1194.

[126] Han, LK; Sumiyoshi, M; Zheng, YN; Okuda, H; Kimura, Y. Anti-obesity action of Salix matsudana leaves (Part 2). Isolation of anti-obesity effectors from polyphenol fractions of Salix matsudana. *Phytother. Res*, 2003 17: 1195-1198.

[127] Lee, EB. Pharmacological studies on Platycodon grandiflorum A. DC. IV. A comparison of experimental pharmacological effects of crude platycodin with clinical indications of platycodi radix *Yakugaku Zasshi*, 1973 93: 1188-1194.

[128] Kim, KS; Ezaki, O; Ikemoto, S; Itakura, H. Effects of Platycodon grandiflorum feeding on serum and liver lipid concentrations in rats with diet-induced hyperlipidemia. *J. Nutr. Sci. Vitaminol. (Tokyo)*, 1995 41: 485-491.

[129] Hiroahi, I; Kauzuo, T; Yohko, Y. Saponins from the roots of Platycodon grandiflorum. Part 1: structure of prosapogenins. *J. Chem. Soc. Perkin. Trans*, 1981: 1928−1933.

[130] Han, L; Zheng, Y; Xu, B; Okuda, H; Kimura, Y. Saponins from Platycodi radix ameliorate high fat diet-induced obesity in mice. *J. Nutr*, 2002 132: 2241-2245.

[131] Han, LK; Xu, BJ; Kimura, Y; Zheng, Y; Okuda, H. Platycodi radix affects lipid metabolism in mice with high fat diet-induced obesity. *J. Nutr*, 2000 130: 2760-2764.

[132] Zhao, HL; Sim, JS; Ha, YW; Kang, SS; Kim, YS. Antiobese and hypolipidemic effects of platycodin saponins in diet-induced obese rats: evidences for lipase inhibition and calorie intake restriction. *Int. J. Obes. (Lond)*, 2005 29: 983-990.

[133] Lee, EB. Pharmacological activities of crude platycodin. *J. Pharmaceut. Soc. Korea*, 1975 19: 164–176.

[134] Han, L; Nose, R; Li, W; Gong, X; Zheng, Y; Yoshikawa, M; Koike, K; Nikaido, T; Okuda, H; Kimura, Y. Reduction of fat storage in mice fed a high-fat diet long term by treatment with saponins prepared from Kochia scoparia fruit. *Phytother. Res*, 2006 20: 877-882.

[135] Qian, XZ. *Colored Illustrations of Chinese Herbs: Part II*. Beijing, People's Health Press; 1996.

[136] Kimura, H; Ogawa, S; Jisaka, M; Kimura, Y; Katsube, T; Yokota, K. Identification of novel saponins from edible seeds of Japanese horse chestnut (Aesculus turbinata Blume) after treatment with wooden ashes and their nutraceutical activity. *J. Pharm. Biomed. Anal.* 2006 41: 1657-1665.

[137] Kimura, H; Ogawa, S; Katsube, T; Jisaka, M; Yokota, K. Antiobese effects of novel saponins from edible seeds of Japanese horse chestnut (Aesculus turbinata BLUME) after treatment with wood ashes. *J. Agric. Food Chem*, 2008 56: 4783-4788.

[138] Hu, JN; Zhu, XM; Han, LK; Saito, M; Sun, Y; Yoshikawa, M; Kimura, Y; Zheng, YN. Anti-obesity effects of escins extracted from the seeds of Aesculus turbinata BLUME (Hippocastanaceae). *Chem. Pharm. Bull. (Tokyo)*, 2008 56: 12-16.

[139] Han, LK; Kimura, Y; Kawashima, M; Takaku, T; Taniyama, T; Hayashi, T; Zheng, YN; Okuda, H. Anti-obesity effects in rodents of dietary teasaponin, a lipase inhibitor. *Int. J. Obes*, 2001 25: 1459-1464.

[140] Muramatsu, K; Fukuyo, M; Hara, Y. Effect of green tea catechins on plasma cholesterol level in cholesterol-fed rats. *J. Nutr. Sci. Vitaminol. (Tokyo)*, 1986 32: 613-622.

[141] Ikeda, I; Imasato, Y; Sasaki, E; Nakayama, M; Nagao, H; Takeo, T; Yayabe, F; Sugano, M. Tea catechins decrease micellar solubility and intestinal absorption of cholesterol in rats. *Biochim. Biophys. Acta*, 1992 1127: 141-146.

[142] Nagao, T; Komine, Y; Soga, S; Meguro, S; Hase, T; Tanaka, Y; Tokimitsu, I. Ingestion of a tea rich in catechins leads to a reduction in body fat and malondialdehyde-modified LDL in men. *Am. J. Clin. Nutr*, 2005 81: 122-129.

[143] Balentine, DA; Wiseman, SA; Bouwens, LC. The chemistry of tea flavonoids. *Crit. Rev. Food Sci. Nutr*, 1997 37: 693-704.

[144] Wolfram, S; Wang, Y; Thielecke, F. Anti-obesity effects of green tea: from bedside to bench. *Mol. Nutr. Food Res*, 2006 50: 176-187.

[145] Thielecke, F; Boschmann, M. The potential role of green tea catechins in the prevention of the metabolic syndrome - A review. *Phytochemistry*, 2009 Epub ahead of printing.

[146] Sano, M; Tabata, M; Suzuki, M; Degawa, M; Miyase, T; Maeda-Yamamoto, M. Simultaneous determination of twelve tea catechins by high-performance liquid chromatography with electrochemical detection. *Analyst*, 2001 126: 816-820.

[147] Mandel, SA; Amit, T; Weinreb, O; Reznichenko, L; Youdim, MB. Simultaneous manipulation of multiple brain targets by green tea catechins: a potential neuroprotective strategy for Alzheimer and Parkinson diseases. *CNS Neurosci. Ther*, 2008 14: 352-365.

[148] Wolfram, S; Raederstorff, D; Wang, Y; Teixeira, SR; Elste, V; Weber, P. TEAVIGO (epigallocatechin gallate) supplementation prevents obesity in rodents by reducing adipose tissue mass. *Ann. Nutr. Metab*, 2005 49: 54-63.

[149] Furuyashiki, T; Nagayasu, H; Aoki, Y; Bessho, H; Hashimoto, T; Kanazawa, K; Ashida, H. Tea catechin suppresses adipocyte differentiation accompanied by down-regulation of PPARgamma2 and C/EBPalpha in 3T3-L1 cells. *Biosci. Biotechnol. Biochem*, 2004 68: 2353-2359.

[150] Hung, PF; Wu, BT; Chen, HC; Chen, YH; Chen, CL; Wu, MH; Liu, HC; Lee, MJ; Kao, YH. Antimitogenic effect of green tea (-)-epigallocatechin gallate on 3T3-L1 preadipocytes depends on the ERK and Cdk2 pathways. *Am. J. Physiol. Cell Physiol*, 2005 288: C1094-1108.

[151] Shimizu, M; Kobayashi, Y; Suzuki, M; Satsu, H; Miyamoto, Y. Regulation of intestinal glucose transport by tea catechins. *Biofactors*, 2000 13: 61-65.

[152] Matsumoto, N; Ishigaki, F; Ishigaki, A; Iwashina, H; Hara, Y. Reduction of blood glucose levels by tea catechin. *Biosci. Biotechnol. Biochem*, 1993 57: 525-527.

[153] Dulloo, AG; Seydoux, J; Girardier, L; Chantre, P; Vandermander, J. Green tea and thermogenesis: interactions between catechin-polyphenols, caffeine and sympathetic activity. *Int. J. Obes. Relat. Metab. Disord*, 2000 24: 252-258.

[154] Borchardt, RT; Huber, JA. Catechol O-methyltransferase. 5. Structure-activity relationships for inhibition by flavonoids. *J. Med. Chem*, 1975 18: 120-122.

[155] Zheng, G; Sayama, K; Okubo, T; Juneja, LR; Oguni, I. Anti-obesity effects of three major components of green tea, catechins, caffeine and theanine, in mice. *In Vivo*, 2004 18: 55-62.

[156] Dulloo, AG; Seydoux, J; Girardier, L. Paraxanthine (metabolite of caffeine) mimics caffeine's interaction with sympathetic control of thermogenesis. *Am. J. Physiol*, 1994 267: E801-E804.

[157] Yoshioka, M; Doucet, E; Drapeau, V; Dionne, I; Tremblay, A. Combined effects of red pepper and caffeine consumption on 24 h energy balance in subjects given free access to foods. *Br. J. Nutr.* 2001 85: 203-211.

[158] Dulloo, AG. Herbal simulation of ephedrine and caffeine in treatment of obesity. *Int. J. Obes. Relat. Metab. Disord*, 2002 26: 590-592.

[159] Jessen, AB; Toubro, S; A, A. Effect of chewing gum containing nicotine and caffeine on energy expenditure and substrate utilization in men. *Am. J. Clin. Nutr*, 2003.

[160] Choo, JJ. Green tea reduces body fat accretion caused by high-fat diet in rats through beta-adrenoceptor activation of thermogenesis in brown adipose tissue. *J. Nutr. Biochem*, 2003 14: 671-676.

[161] Hasegawa, N; Yamda, N; Mori, M. Powdered green tea has antilipogenic effect on Zucker rats fed a high-fat diet. *Phytother. Res*, 2003 17: 477-480.

[162] Ashida, H; Furuyashiki, T; Nagayasu, H; Bessho, H; Sakakibara, H; Hashimoto, T; Kanazawa, K. Anti-obesity actions of green tea: possible involvements in modulation of the glucose uptake system and suppression of the adipogenesis-related transcription factors. *Biofactors*, 2004 22: 135-140.

[163] Hase, T; Komine, Y; Meguro, S; Takeda, Y; Takahashi, H; Matusi, Y. Anti-obesity effects of tea catechins in humans. *J. Oleo. Sci*, 2001 50: 599-605.

[164] Tsuchida, T; Itakura, H; Nakamura, H. Reduction of body fat in humans by long-term ingestion of catechins. *Prog. Med*, 2002 22: 2189-2203.

[165] Kovacs, EM; Mela, DJ. Metabolically active functional food ingredients for weight control. *Obes. Rev*, 2006 7: 59-78.

[166] Auvichayapat, P; Prapochanung, M; Tunkamnerdthai, O; Sripanidkulchai, BO; Auvichayapat, N; Thinkhamrop, B; Kunhasura, S; Wongpratoom, S; Sinawat, S; Hongprapas, P. Effectiveness of green tea

on weight reduction in obese Thais: A randomized, controlled trial. *Physiol. Behav*, 2008 93: 486-491.

[167] Nagao, T; Hase, T; Tokimitsu, I. A green tea extract high in catechins reduces body fat and cardiovascular risks in humans. *Obesity (Silver Spring)*, 2007 15: 1473-1483.

[168] Maki, KC; Reeves, MS; Farmer, M; Yasunaga, K; Matsuo, N; Katsuragi, Y; Komikado, M; Tokimitsu, I; Wilder, D; Jones, F; Blumberg, JB; Cartwright, Y. Green tea catechin consumption enhances exercise-induced abdominal fat loss in overweight and obese adults. *J. Nutr*, 2009 139: 264-270.

[169] Diepvens, K; Kovacs, EM; Vogels, N; Westerterp-Plantenga, MS. Metabolic effects of green tea and of phases of weight loss. *Physiol. Behav*, 2006 87: 185-191.

[170] Chantre, P; Lairon, D. Recent findings of green tea extract AR25 (Exolise) and its activity for the treatment of obesity. *Phytomedicine*, 2002 9: 3-8.

[171] Dulloo, AG; Duret, C; Rohrer, D; Girardier, L; Mensi, N; Fathi, M; Chantre, P; Vandermander, J. Efficacy of a green tea extract rich in catechin polyphenols and caffeine in increasing 24-h energy expenditure and fat oxidation in humans. *Am. J. Clin. Nutr*, 1999 70: 1040-1045.

[172] Rumpler, W; Seale, J; Clevidence, B; Judd, J; Wiley, E; Yamamoto, S; Komatsu, T; Sawaki, T; Ishikura, Y; Hosoda, K. Oolong tea increases metabolic rate and fat oxidation in men. *J. Nutr*, 2001 131: 2848-2852.

[173] Rudelle, S; Ferruzzi, MG; Cristiani, I; Moulin, J; Mace, K; Acheson, KJ; Tappy, L. Effect of a thermogenic beverage on 24-hour energy metabolism in humans. *Obesity (Silver Spring)*, 2007 15: 349-355.

[174] Belza, A; Toubro, S; A, A. The effect of caffeine, green tea and tyrosine on thermogenesis and energy intake. *Eur. J. Clin. Nutr*, 2007 Epub ahead of print.

[175] del Castillo, MD; Ames, JM; Gordon, MH. Effect of roasting on the antioxidant activity of coffee brews. *J. Agric. Food Chem*, 2002 50: 3698-3703.

[176] Suzuki, A; Kagawa, D; Ochiai, R; Tokimitsu, I; Saito, I. Green coffee bean extract and its metabolites have a hypotensive effect in spontaneously hypertensive rats. *Hypertens Res*, 2002 25: 99-107.

[177] Arion, WJ; Canfield, WK; Ramos, FC; Schindler, PW; Burger, HJ; Hemmerle, H; Schubert, G; Below, P; Herling, AW. Chlorogenic acid and hydroxynitrobenzaldehyde: new inhibitors of hepatic glucose 6-phosphatase. *Arch. Biochem. Biophys*, 1997 339: 315-322.

[178] Shimoda, H; Seki, E; Aitani, M. Inhibitory effect of green coffee bean extract on fat accumulation and body weight gain in mice. *BMC Complement Altern. Med*, 2006 6: 9.

[179] Thom, E. The effect of chlorogenic acid enriched coffee on glucose absorption in healthy volunteers and its effect on body mass when used long-term in overweight and obese people. *J. Int. Med. Res*, 2007 35: 900-908.

[180] Herling, AW; Burger, HJ; Schwab, D; Hemmerle, H; Below, P; Schubert, G. Pharmacodynamic profile of a novel inhibitor of the hepatic glucose-6-phosphatase system. *Am. J. Physiol*, 1998 274: G1087-1093.

[181] Pellati, F; Benvenuti, S; Melegari, M; Firenzuoli, F. Determination of adrenergic agonists from extracts and herbal products of Citrus aurantium L. var. amara by LC. *J. Pharm. Biomed. Anal*, 2002 29: 1113-1119.

[182] Preuss, HG; DiFerdinando, D; Bagchi, M; Bagchi, D. Citrus aurantium as a thermogenic, weight-reduction replacement for ephedra: an overview. *J. Med*, 2002 33: 247-264.

[183] Haaz, S; Fontaine, KR; Cutter, G; Limdi, N; Perumean-Chaney, S; Allison, DB. Citrus aurantium and synephrine alkaloids in the treatment of overweight and obesity: an update. *Obes. Rev*, 2006 7: 79-88.

[184] Astrup, A. Thermogenic drugs as a strategy for treatment of obesity. *Endocrine*, 2000 13: 207-212.

[185] National Toxicology Program. NTP toxicology and carcinogenesis studies of ephedrine sulfate (CAS, 134-72-5) in F344/N rats and B6C3F1 mice (Feed Studies). *Natl. Toxicol. Program Tech. Rep. Series* 1986 307: 1-186.

[186] Mooney, RA; McDonald, JM. Effect of phenylephrine on lipolysis in rat adipocytes: no evidence for an alpha-adrenergic mechanism. *Int. J. Biochem*, 1984 16: 55-59.

[187] Yeh, SY. Comparative anorectic effects of metaraminol and phenylephrine in rats. *Physiol. Behav*, 1999 68: 227-234.

[188] Desfaits, AC; Lafond, J; Savard, R. The effects of a selective alpha-1 adrenergic blockade on the activity of adipose tissue lipoprotein lipase in female hamsters. *Life Sci*, 1995 57: 705-713.

[189] Calapai, G; Firenzuoli, F; Saitta, A; Squadrito, F; Arlotta, M; Costantino, G; Inferrera, G. Antiobesity and cardiovascular toxic effects of Citrus aurantium extracts in the rat: a preliminary report. *Fitoterapia*, 1999 70: 586-592.

[190] Attele, AS; Wu, JA; Yuan, CS. Ginseng pharmacology: multiple constituents and multiple actions. *Biochem. Pharmacol*, 1999 58: 1685-1693.

[191] Yuan, CS; Wu, JA; Osinski, J. Ginsenoside variability in American ginseng samples. *Am. J. Clin. Nutr*, 2002 75: 600-601.

[192] Liu, W; Zheng, Y; Han, L; Wang, H; Saito, M; Ling, M; Kimura, Y; Feng, Y. Saponins (Ginsenosides) from stems and leaves of Panax quinquefolium prevented high-fat diet-induced obesity in mice. *Phytomedicine*, 2008 15: 1140-1145.

[193] Etou, H; Sakata, T; Fujimoto, K; Terada, K; Yoshimatsu, H; Ookuma, K; Hayashi, T; Arichi, S. Ginsenoside-Rb1 as a suppressor in central modulation of feeding in the rat. *Nippon Yakurigaku Zasshi*, 1988 91: 9-15.

[194] Cooper, SJ; Al-Naser, HA; Clifton, PG. The anorectic effect of the selective dopamine D1-receptor agonist A-77636 determined by meal pattern analysis in free-feeding rats. *Eur. J. Pharmacol*, 2006 532: 253-257.

[195] Kim, JH; Kang, SA; Han, SM; Shim, I. Comparison of the antiobesity effects of the protopanaxadiol- and protopanaxatriol-type saponins of red ginseng. *Phytother. Res*, 2009 23: 78-85.

[196] Fredholm, BB; Bättig, K; Holmén, J; Nehlig, A; Zvartau, EE. Actions of caffeine in the brain with special reference to factors that contribute to its widespread use. *Pharmacol. Rev*, 1999 51: 83-133.

[197] Quarta, D; Borycz, J; Solinas, M; Patkar, K; Hockemeyer, J; Ciruela, F; Lluis, C; Franco, R; Woods, AS; Goldberg, SR; Ferré, S. Adenosine receptor-mediated modulation of dopamine release in the nucleus accumbens depends on glutamate neurotransmission and N-methyl-D-aspartate receptor stimulation. *J. Neurochem*, 2004 91: 873-880.

[198] Krugel, U; Schraft, T; Regenthal, R; Illes, P; Kittner, H. Purinergic modulation of extracellular glutamate levels in the nucleus accumbens in vivo. *Int. J. Dev. Neurosci*, 2004 22: 565-570.

[199] De Luca, MA; Bassareo, V; Bauer, A; Di Chiara, G. Caffeine and accumbens shell dopamine. *J. Neurochem*, 2007 103: 157-163.

[200] Arolfo, MP; Yao, L; Gordon, AS; Diamond, I; Janak, PH. Ethanol operant self-administration in rats is regulated by adenosine A2 receptors. *Alcohol. Clin. Exp. Res*, 2004 28: 1308-1316.

[201] Schiffman, SS; Diaz, C; Beeker, TG. Caffeine intensifies taste of certain sweeteners: role of adenosine receptor. *Pharmacol. Biochem. Behav*, 1986 24: 429-432.

[202] Schiffman, SS; Gill, JM; Diaz, C. Methyl xanthines enhance taste: evidence for modulation of taste by adenosine receptor. *Pharmacol. Biochem. Behav*, 1985 22: 195-203.

[203] Cheung, WT; Lee, CM; Ng, TB. Potentiation of the anti-lipolytic effect of 2-chloroadenosine after chronic caffeine treatment. *Pharmacology*, 1988 36: 331-339.

[204] Muroyama, K; Murosaki, S; Yamamoto, Y; Odaka, H; Chung, HC; Miyoshi, M. Anti-obesity effects of a mixture of thiamin, arginine, caffeine, and citric acid in non-insulin dependent diabetic KK mice. *J. Nutr. Sci. Vitaminol (Tokyo)*, 2003 49: 56-63.

[205] Pettenuzzo, L; Noschang, C; von Pozzer Toigo, E; Fachin, A; Vendite, D; Dalmaz, C. Effects of chronic administration of caffeine and stress on feeding behavior of rats. *Physiol. Behav*, 2008 95: 295-301.

[206] Kelley, AE; Baldo, BA; Pratt, WE; Will, MJ. Corticostriatal-hypothalamic circuitry and food motivation: Integration of energy, action and reward. *Physiol. Behav*, 2005 86: 773-795.

[207] Meister, B. Neurotransmitters in key neurons of the hypothalamus that regulate feeding behavior and body weight. *Physiol. Behav*, 2007 92: 263-271.

[208] Acquas, E; Tanda, G; Di Chiara, G. Differential effects of caffeine on dopamine and acetylcholine transmission in brain areas of drug-naive and caffeine-pretreated rats. *Neuropsychopharmacology*, 2002 27: 182-193.

[209] Carney, JM. Effects of caffeine, theophylline and theobromine on scheduled controlled responding in rats. *Br. J. Pharmacol*, 1982 75: 451-454.

[210] Chen, MD; Lin, WH; Song, YM; Lin, PY; Ho, LT. Effect of caffeine on the levels of brain serotonin and catecholamine in the genetically obese mice. *Zhonghua Yi Xue Za Zhi (Taipei)*, 1994 53: 257-261.

[211] Halford, JC; Blundell, JE. Pharmacology of appetite suppression. *Prog. Drug Res*, 2000 54: 25-58.

[212] Diepvens, K; Westerterp, KR; Westerterp-Plantenga, MS. Obesity and thermogenesis related to the consumption of caffeine, ephedrine, capsaicin, and green tea. *Am. J. Physiol. Regul. Integr. Comp. Physiol*, 2007 292: R77-R85.

[213] Astrup, A; Breum, L; Toubro, S; Hein, P; Quaade, F. The effect and safety of an ephedrine/caffeine compound compared to ephedrine, caffeine and placebo in obese subjects on an energy restricted diet. A double blind trial. *Int. J. Obes. Relat. Metab. Disord*, 1992 16: 269-277.

[214] Pasman, WJ; Westerterp-Plantenga, MS; Saris, WH. The effectiveness of long-term supplementation of carbohydrate, chromium, fibre and caffeine on weight maintenance. *Int. J. Obes. Relat. Metab. Disord*, 1997 21: 1143-1151.

[215] Westerterp-Plantenga, MS; Lejeune, MP; Kovacs, EM. Body weight loss and weight maintenance in relation to habitual caffeine intake and green tea supplementation. *Obes. Res*, 2005 13: 1195-1204.

[216] Tremblay, A; Masson, E; Leduc, S; A, H; Despres, JP. Caffeine reduces spontaneous energy intake in men but not in women. *Nutr. Res*, 1988 8: 553-558.

[217] Racotta, S; Leblanc, J; Richard, D. The effect of caffeine on food intake in rats: involvement of corticotropin-releasing factor and the sympatho-adrenal system. *Pharmacol. Biochem. Behav*, 1994 48: 887-892.

[218] Comer, SD; Haney, M; W, FR; Fischman, MW. Effects of caffeine withdrawal on humans living in a residential laboratory. *Exp. Clin. Psychopharmacol*, 1997 5: 399-403.

[219] Jessen, A; Buemann, B; Toubro, S; Skovgaard, IM; Astrup, A. The appetite-suppressant effect of nicotine is enhanced by caffeine. *Diab. Ob. Metab*, 2005 7: 327-333.

[220] Lopez-Garcia, E; van Dam, RM; Rajpathak, S; Willett, WC; Manson, JE; Hu, FB. Changes in caffeine intake and long-term weight change in men and women. *Am. J. Clin. Nutr*, 2006 83: 674-680.

[221] Jung, RT; Shetty, PS; James, WP; Barrand, MA; Callingham, BA. Caffeine: its effect on catecholamines and metabolism in lean and obese humans. *Clin. Sci. (Lond)*, 1981 60: 527-535.

[222] Hollands, MA; Arch, JR; Cawthorne, MA. A simple apparatus for comparative measurements of energy expenditure in human subjects: the thermic effect of caffeine. *Am. J. Clin. Nutr*, 1981 34: 2291-2294.

[223] Graham, TE. Caffeine and exercise: metabolism, endurance and performance. *Sports Med*, 2001 31: 785-807.

[224] Acheson, KJ; Zahorska-Markiewicz, B; Pittet, P; Anantharaman, K; Jequier, E. Caffeine and coffee: their influence on metabolic rate and substrate utilization in normal weight and obese individuals. *Am. J. Clin. Nutr*, 1980 33: 989-997.

[225] Dulloo, AG. Ephedrine, xanthines and prostaglandin-inhibitors: actions and interactions in the stimulation of thermogenesis. *Int. J. Obes. Relat. Metab. Disord*, 1993 17 S35-S40.

[226] Astrup, A; Toubro, S. Thermogenic, metabolic, and cardiovascular responses to ephedrine and caffeine in man. *Int. J. Obes. Relat. Metab. Disord*, 1993 17 S41-S43.

[227] Astrup, A; Toubro, S; Cannon, S; Hein, P; Breum, L; Madsen, J. Caffeine: a double-blind, placebo-controlled study of its thermogenic, metabolic, and cardiovascular effects in healthy volunteers. *Am. J. Clin. Nutr*, 1990 51: 759-767.

[228] Yoshida, T; Sakane, N; Umekawa, T; Kondo, M. Relationship between basal metabolic rate, thermogenic response to caffeine, and body weight loss following combined low calorie and exercise treatment in obese women. *Int. J. Obes. Relat. Metab. Disord*, 1994 18: 345-350.

[229] Haller, CA; Jacob, Pr; Benowitz, N. Enhanced stimulant and metabolic effects of combined ephedrine and caffeine. *Clin. Pharmacol. Ther*, 2004 75: 259-273.

[230] Taylor, P. Ganglionic stimulating and blocking agents, In: Oillman, AG, et al., editor. *The Pharmacological Basis of Therapeutics*. New York: McMiilan; 1985.

[231] Perkins, KA; Epstein, LH; Stiller, RL; Fernstrom, MH; Sexton, JE; Jacob, RG; Solberg, R. Acute effects of nicotine on hunger and caloric intake in smokers and nonsmokers. *Psychopharmacology*, 1991 103: 103-109.

[232] Albanes, D; Jones, DY; Micozzi, MS; Mattson, ME. Associations between smoking and body weight in the U.S. population: analysis of NHANES II. *Am. J. Public Health*, 1987 77: 439-444.

[233] Jo, YH; Talmage, DA; Role, LW. Nicotinic receptor-mediated effects on appetite and food intake. *J. Neurobiol*, 2002 53: 618-632.

[234] Grunberg, NE; Bowen, DJ; Winders, SE. Effects of nicotine on body weight and food consumption in female rats. *Psychopharmacology (Berl)*, 1986 90: 101-105.

[235] Klesges, RC; Meyers, AW; Klesges, LM; La Vasque, ME. Smoking, body weight, and their effects on smoking behavior: a comprehensive review of the literature. *Psychol. Bull*, 1989 106: 204-230.

[236] Pomerleau, CS. Issues for women who wish to stop smoking, In: Seidman, DF and Covey, LS, editor. *Helping the hard-core smoker*. London: Lawrence Erlbaum; 1999;p. 73-91.

[237] Pomerleau, CS; Pomerleau, OF; Namenek, RJ; Mehringer, AM. Short-term weight gain in abstaining women smokers. *J. Subst. Abuse Treat*, 2000 18: 339-342.

[238] Dallosso, HM; James, WP. The role of smoking in the regulation of energy balance. *Int. J. Obes*, 1984 8: 365-375.

[239] Stamford, BA; Matter, S; Fell, RD; Papanek, P. Effects of smoking cessation on weight gain, metabolic rate, caloric consumption, and blood lipids. *Am. J. Clin. Nutr*, 1986 43: 486-494.

[240] Sztalryd, C; Hamilton, J; Horowitz, BA; Johnson, P; Kraemer, FB. Alterations of lipolysis and lipoprotein lipase in chronically nicotine-treated rats. *Am. J. Physiol*, 1996 270: E215-E223.

[241] Ashakumary, L; Vijayammal, PL. Effect of nicotine on lipoprotein metabolism in rats. *Lipids*, 1997 32: 311-315.

[242] Arai, K; Kim, K; Kaneko, K; Iketani, M; Otagiri, A; Yamauchi, N; Shibasaki, T. Nicotine infusion alters leptin and uncoupling protein 1 mRNA expression in adipose tissues of rats. *Am. J. Physiol. Endocrinol. Metab*, 2001 280: E867-E876.

[243] Sanigorski, A; Fahey, R; Cameron-Smith, D; Collier, GR. Nicotine treatment decreases food intake and body weight via a leptin-independent pathway in Psammomys obesus. *Diabetes Obes. Metab*, 2002 4: 346-350.

[244] Winders, SE; Grunberg, NE. Effects of nicotine on body weight, food consumption and body composition in male rats. *Life Sci*, 1990 46: 1523-1530.

[245] Chen, H; Hansen, MJ; Jones, JE; Vlahos, R; Bozinovski, S; Anderson, GP; Morris, MJ. Regulation of hypothalamic NPY by diet and smoking. *Peptides*, 2007 28: 384-389.

[246] Kane, JK; Parker, SL; Li, MD. Hypothalamic orexin-A binding sites are downregulated by chronic nicotine treatment in the rat. *Neurosci. Lett*, 2001 298: 1-4.

[247] Yang, ZJ; Blaha, V; Meguid, MM; Oler, A; Miyata, G. Infusion of nicotine into the LHA enhances dopamine and 5-HT release and suppresses food intake. *Pharmacol. Biochem. Behav*, 1999 64: 155-159.

[248] Miyata, G; Meguid, MM; Fetissov, SO; Torelli, GF; Kim, HJ. Nicotine's effect on hypothalamic neurotransmitters and appetite regulation. *Surgery*, 1999 126: 255-263.

[249] Mifsud, JC; Hernandez, L; Hoebel, BG. Nicotine infused into the nucleus accumbens increases synaptic dopamine as measured by in vivo microdialysis. *Brain Res*, 1989 478: 365-367.

[250] Nisell, M; Nomikos, GG; Svensson, TH. Infusion of nicotine in the ventral tegmental area or the nucleus accumbens of the rat differentially

affects accumbal dopamine release. *Pharmacol. Toxicol*, 1994 75: 348-352.

[251] Zarrindast, MR; Oveisi, MR. Effects of monoamine receptor antagonists on nicotine-induced hypophagia in the rat. *Eur. J. Pharmacol*, 1997 321: 157-162.

[252] Williamson, DF; Madans, J; Anda, RF; Kleinman, JC; Giovino, GA; Byers, T. Smoking cessation and severity of weight gain in a national cohort. *N. Engl. J. Med*, 1991 324: 739-745.

[253] Shimokata, H; Muller, DC; Andres, R. Studies in the distribution of body fat. III. Effects of cigarette smoking. *JAMA*, 1989 261: 1169-1173.

[254] Flegal, KM; Troiano, RP; Pamuk, ER; Kuczmarski, RJ; Campbell, SM. The influence of smoking cessation on the prevalence of overweight in the United States. *N. Engl. J. Med*, 1995 333: 1165-1170.

[255] Huot, I; Paradis, G; Ledoux, M. Quebec Heart Health Demonstration Project Research Group. Factors associated with overweight and obesity in Quebec adults. *Int. J. Obes. Relat. Metab. Disord*, 2004 28: 766-774.

[256] Blaha, V; Yang, ZJ; Meguid, M; Chai, JK; Zadak, Z. Systemic nicotine administration suppresses food intake via reduced meal sizes in both male and female rats. *Acta Med*, 1998 41: 167-173.

[257] Miyata, G; Meguid, MM; Varma, M; Fetissov, SO; Kim, HJ. Nicotine alters the usual reciprocity between meal size and meal number in female rat. *Physiol. Behav*, 2001 74: 169-176.

[258] Bray, GA. Reciprocal relation of food intake and sympathetic activity: experimental observations and clinical implications. *Int. J. Obes. Relat. Metab. Disord*, 2000 24: S8-S17.

[259] Zhang, L; Meguid, MM; Miyata, G; Varma, M; Fetissov, SO. Role of hypothalamic monoamines in nicotine-induced anorexia in menopausal rats. *Surgery*, 2001 130: 133-142.

[260] McNair, E; Bryson, R. Effects of nicotine on weight change and food consumption in rats. *Pharmacol. Biochem. Behav*, 1983 18: 341-344.

[261] Grunberg, NE; Bowen, DJ; Morse, DE. Effects of nicotine on body weight and food consumption in rats. *Psychopharmacology (Berl)*, 1984 83: 93-98.

[262] Schechter, MD; Cook, PG. Nicotine-induced weight loss in rats without an effect on appetite. *Eur. J. Pharmacol*, 1976 38: 63-69.

[263] Morgan, MM; Ellison, G. Different effects of chronic nicotine treatment regimens on body weight and tolerance in the rat. *Psychopharmacology. (Berl)*, 1987 91: 236-238.

[264] Wager-Srdar, SA; Levine, AS; Morley, JE; Hoidal, JR; Niewoehner, DE. Effects of cigarette smoke and nicotine on feeding and energy. *Physiol. Behav*, 1984 32: 389-395.

[265] Grunberg, NE; Bowen, DJ; Maycock, VA; Nespor, SM. The importance of sweet taste and caloric content in the effects of nicotine on specific food consumption. *Psychopharmacology (Berl)*, 1985 87: 198-203.

[266] Filozof, C; Fernandez Pinilla, MC; Fernandez-Cruz, A. Smoking cessation and weight gain. *Obes. Rev*, 2004 5: 95-103.

[267] Gross, J; Stitzer, ML; Maldonado, J. Nicotine replacement: effects of postcessation weight gain. *J. Consult. Clin. Psychol*, 1989 57: 87-92.

[268] Allen, SS; Hatsukami, D; Brintnell, DM; Bade, T. Effect of nicotine replacement therapy on post-cessation weight gain and nutrient intake: a randomized controlled trial of postmenopausal female smokers. *Addict. Behav*, 2005 30: 1273-1280.

[269] Murray, CD; Le Roux, CW; Emmanuel, AV; Halket, JM; Przyborowska, AM; Kamm, MA; Murray-Lyon, IM. The effect of Khat (Catha edulis) as an appetite suppressant is independent of ghrelin and PYY secretion. *Appetite*, 2008 51: 747-750.

[270] Le Bras, M; Fretillere, Y. Les aspects mrdicaux de la consommation habituelle du Cath. *Mdd. trop*, 1965 25: 720-731.

[271] Halbach, H. Medical aspects of the chewing of khat leaves. *Bull. Wld. Hlth. Org*, 1972 47: 21-29.

[272] Zelger, JL; Carlini, EA. Anorexigenic effects of two amines obtained from Catha edulis Forsk. (Khat) in rats. *Pharmacol. Biochem. Behav*, 1980 12: 701-705.

[273] Toennes, SW; Harder, S; Schramm, M; Niess, C; Kauert, GF. Pharmacokinetics of cathinone, cathine and norephedrine after the chewing of khat leaves. *Br. J. Clin. Pharmacol*, 2003 56: 125-130.

[274] Zelger, JL; Schorno, HX; Carlini, EA. Behavioural effects of cathinone, an amine obtained from Catha edulis Forsk.: comparisons with amphetamine, norpseudoephedrine, apomorphine and nomifensine. *Bull. Narc*, 1980 32: 67-81.

[275] Eisenberg, MS; Maher, TJ; Silverman, HI. A comparison of the effects of phenylpropanolamine, d-amphetamine and d-norpseudoephedrine on open-field locomotion and food intake in the rat. *Appetite*, 1987 9: 31-37.

[276] Heymann, TD; Bhupulan, A; Zureikat, NE; Bomanji, J; Drinkwater, C; Giles, P; Murray-Lyon, IM. Khat chewing delays gastric emptying of a semi-solid meal. *Aliment Pharmacol. Ther*, 1995 9: 81-83.

[277] Van Beek, TA; Verpoorte, R; Svendsen, AB; Leeuwenberg, AJ; Bisset, NG. Tabernaemontana L. (Apocynaceae): a review of its taxonomy, phytochemistry, ethnobotany and pharmacology. *J. Ethnopharmacol*, 1984 10: 1-156.

[278] Bruyns, P. A revision of hoodia and lavrania (Asclepidaceae-Stapeliaeae Botanische Jahrbucher:fuer). *Syst. Pflanzenges Pflanzengeogr*, 1993 115: 145-270.

[279] van Heerden, FR. Hoodia gordonii: A natural appetite suppressant. *J. Ethnopharmacol*, 2008 119 434-437.

[280] Van Heerden, FR; Horak, RM; Learmonth, RA; Maharaj, V; Whittal, RD, *Pharmaceutical compositions having appetite-suppressant activity*. 1998.

[281] Van Heerden, FR; Horak, RM; Maharaj, VJ; Vleggaar, R; Senabe, JV; Gunning, PJ. An appetite suppressant from Hoodia species. *Phytochemistry*, 2007 68: 2545-2553.

[282] Tulp, OL; Harbi, NA; Mihalov, J; DerMarderosian, A. Effect of Hoodia plant on food intake and body weight in lean and obese LA/Ntul//-cp rats. *FASEB J*, 2001 15: A404.

[283] Phytopharm open offer and placing prospectus 080228. 2008: 1-129.

[284] MacLean, DB; Luo, LG. Increased ATP content/production in the hypothalamus may be a signal for energy-sensing of satiety: studies of the anorectic mechanism of a plant steroidal glycoside. *Brain Res*, 2004 1020: 1-11.

[285] MacLean, DB. Abrogation of peripheral cholecystokinin-satiety in the capsaicin treated rat. *Regul. Pept*, 1985 11: 321-333.

[286] Laddha, KS, *Medicinal Natural Products Research Laboratory*, University of Mumbai: Mumbai, India.

[287] *Wealth of India. A Dictionary of Indian Raw Materials and Industrial Products*. 1992. p. 266-267.

[288] Bader, A; Braca, A; De Tommasi, Na; Morelli, I. Further constituents from Caralluma negevensis. *Phytochemistry*, 2003 62: 1277-1281.

[289] Preuss, HG; Bagchi, D; Bagchi, M; Rao, CV; Dey, DK; Satyanarayana, S. Effects of a natural extract of (-)-hydroxycitric acid (HCA-SX) and a combination of HCA-SX plus niacin-bound chromium and Gymnema sylvestre extract on weight loss. *Diabetes Obes Metab*, 2004 6: 171-180.

[290] Preuss, HG, *Report on the Safety of Caralluma Fimbriata and its Extract*. 2004: Washington, D C.

[291] Kuriyan, R; Raj, T; Srinivas, SK; Vaz, M; Rajendran, R; Kurpad, AV. Effect of Caralluma fimbriata extract on appetite, food intake and

anthropometry in adult Indian men and women. *Appetite*, 2007 48: 338-344.

[292] Roberts, SB; Heyman, MB. Dietary composition and obesity: do we need to look beyond dietary fat? *J. Nutr*, 2000 130: 267S.

[293] Agarwal, KC; Parks, REJ. Forskolin: a potential antimetastatic agent. *Int. J. Cancer*, 1983 32: 801-804.

[294] Caprioli, J; Sears, M. Forskolin lowers intraocular pressure in rabbits, monkeys, and man. *Lancet*, 1983 1: 958-960.

[295] Burns, TW; Langley, PE; Terry, BE; Bylund, DB; Forte, LRJ. Comparative effects of forskolin and isoproterenol on the cyclic AMP content of human adipocytes. *Life Sci*, 1987 40: 145-154.

[296] Litosch, I; Hudson, TH; Mills, I; Li, SY; Fain, JN. Forskolin as an activator of cyclic AMP accumulation and lipolysis in rat adipocytes. *Mol. Pharmacol*, 1982 22: 109-115.

[297] Henderson, S; Magu, B; Rasmussen, C; Lancaster, S; Kerksick, C; Smith, P; Melton, C; Cowan, P; Greenwood, M; Earnest, C; Almada, A; Milnor, P; Magrans, T; Bowden, R; Ounpraseuth, S; Thomas, A; Kreider, RB. Effects of coleus forskohlii supplementation on body composition and hematological profiles in mildly overweight women. *J. Int. Soc. Sports Nutr*, 2005 2: 54-62.

[298] Gaoni, Y; Mechoulam, R. Isolation, structure and partial synthesis of an active constituent of hashish. *J. Am. Chem Soc*, 1964 86: 1646.

[299] Woelkart, K; Salo-Ahen, OM; Bauer, R. CB receptor ligands from plants. *Curr. Top Med. Chem*, 2008 8: 173-186.

[300] Foltin, RW; Brady, JV; Fischman, MW. Behavioral analysis of marijuana effects on food intake in humans. *Pharmacol. Biochem. Behav*, 1986 25: 577-582.

[301] Foltin, RW; Fischman, MW; Byrne, MF. Effects of smoked marijuana on food intake and body weight of humans living in a residential laboratory. *Appetite*, 1988 11: 1-14.

[302] Haney, M; Rabkin, J; Gunderson, E; Foltin, RW. Dronabinol and marijuana in HIV+ marijuana smokers: acute effects on caloric intake and mood. *Psychopharmacology (Berl)*, 2005 181: 170-178.

[303] Hart, CL; Ward, AS; Haney, M; Comer, SD; Foltin, RW; Fischman, MW. Comparison of smoked marijuana and oral D9-tetrahydrocannbinol in humans. *Psychopharmacology (Berl)*, 2002 164: 407-415.

[304] Haney, M; Ward, AS; Comer, SD; Foltin, RW; Fischman, MW. Abstinence symptoms following oral THC administration to humans. *Psychopharmacology (Berl)*, 1999 141: 385-394.

[305] Haney, M; Gunderson, EW; Rabkin, J; Hart, CL; Vosburg, SK; Comer, SD; Foltin, RW. Dronabinol and marijuana in HIV-positive marijuana smokers. Caloric intake, mood, and sleep. *J. Acquir. Immune Defic. Syndr*, 2007 45: 545-554.

[306] Abel, EL. Effects of marijuana on the solution of anagrams, memory and appetite. *Nature*, 1971 231: 260-261.

[307] Hollister, LE. Hunger and appetite after single doses of marihuana, alcohol, and dextroamphetamine. *Clin. Pharmacol. Ther*, 1971 12: 44-49.

[308] Huestis, MA; Gorelick , DA; Heishman, SJ; Preston, KL; Nelson, RA; Moolchan, ET; Frank, RA. Blockade of effects of smoked marijuana by the CB1 selective cannabinoid receptor antagonist SR141716. *Arch. Gen. Psychiatry*, 2001 58: 322-328.

[309] Regelson, W; Butler, JR; Schultz, J. Delta-9-tetrahydrocannabinol as an effective antidepressant and appetitestimulating agent in advanced cancer patients, In: Braude, M and Szara, S, editor. *The Pharmacology of Marijuana*. New York:: Raven Press; 1976;p. 763-776.

[310] Beal, JE; Olson, R; Laubenstein, L; Morales, JO; Bellman, P; Yangco, B; Lefkowitz, L; Plasse, TF; Shepard, KV. Dronabinol as a treatment for anorexia associated with weight loss in patients with AIDS. *J. Pain Symptom Manage*, 1995 10: 89-97.

[311] Plasse, TF; Gorter, RW; Krasnow, SH; Lane, M; Shepard, KV; Wadleigh, RG. Recent clinical experience with dronabinol. *Pharmacol. Biochem. Behav*, 1991 40: 695-700.

[312] Struwe, M; Kaempfer, S; Geiger, C; Pavia, A; Plasse, T; Shepard, K; Ries, K; Evans, T. Effect of dronabinol on nutritional status in HIV infection. *Ann. Pharmacother*, 1993 27: 827-831.

[313] Kirkham, TC; Rogers, EK; Tucci, S, *Eating stimulated by intra-PVN infusion of the endocannabinoid 2-AG is reversed by opioid receptor blockade*, in *Society for Neuroscience 35th Annual Meeting*. 2005: Washington USA. p. 533.15.

[314] Williams, CM; Kirkham, TC. Reversal of delta 9-THC hyperphagia by SR141716 and naloxone but not dexfenfluramine. *Pharmacol. Biochem. Behav*, 2002 7: 333-340.

[315] Brown, JE; Kassouny, M; Cross, JK. Kinetic studies of food intake and sucrose solution preference by rats treated with low doses of delta9-tetrahydrocannabinol. *Behav. Biol*, 1977 20: 104-110.

[316] Anderson-Baker, WC; McLaughlin, CL; Baile, CA. Oral and hypothalamic injections of barbiturates, benzodiazepines and

cannabinoids and food intake in rats. *Pharmacol. Biochem. Behav*, 1979 11: 487-491.

[317] Williams, CM; Rogers, PJ; Kirkham, TC. Hyperphagia in pre-fed rats following oral delta9-THC. *Physiol. Behav*, 1998 65: 343-346.

[318] Williams, CM; Kirkham, TC. Anandamide induces overeating: mediation by central cannabinoid (CB1) receptors. *Psychopharmacology*, 1999 143: 315-317.

[319] Williams, CM; Kirkham, TC. Reversal of cannabinoid hyperphagia by naloxone but not dexfenfluramine. *Appetite*, 2000 35: 317.

[320] Williams, CM; Kirkham, TC. Observational analysis of feeding induced by Delta9-THC and anandamide. *Physiol. Behav*, 2002 76: 241-250.

[321] Avraham, Y; Ben-Shushan, D; Brener, A; Zolotarev, O; Okon, O; Fink, N; Katz, V; Berry, EM. Very low dose of tetrahydrocannabinol (THC) improves food consumption and cognitive function in an animal model of anorexia nervosa. *Pharmacol. Biochem. Behav*, 2004 77: 657-684.

[322] Cooper, S. Endocannabinoids and food consumption: comparisons with benzodiazepine and opioid palatability-dependent appetite. *Eur. J. Pharmacol*, 2004 500: 37-49.

[323] Jarrett, MM; Limebeer, CL; Parker, LA. Effect of delta9-tetrahydrocannabinol on sucrose palatability as measured by the taste reactivity test. *Physiol. Behav*, 2005 86: 475-479.

[324] Kirkham, TC. Endocannabinoids in the regulation of appetite and body weight. *Behav. Pharmacol*, 2005 16: 297-313.

[325] Koch, JE; Matthews, SM. Delta9-tetrahydrocannabinol stimulates palatable food intake in Lewis rats: effects of peripheral and central administration. *Nutr. Neurosci*, 2001 4: 179-187.

[326] Higgs, S; Williams, C; Kirkham, T. Cannabinoid influences on palatability: microstructural analysis of sucrose drinking after delta(9)-tetrahydrocannabinol, anandamide, 2-arachidonoyl glycerol and SR141716. *Psychopharmacology*, 2003 165: 370-377.

[327] Mahler, SV; Smith, KS; Berridge, KC. Endocannabinoid hedonic hotspot for sensory pleasure: anandamide in nucleus accumbens shell enhances 'liking' of a sweet reward. *Neuropsychopharmacology*, 2007 32: 2267-2278.

[328] Berridge, KC; Robinson, TE. Parsing reward. *Trends Neurosci*, 2003 26: 507-513.

[329] van Wyk, BE; Albrecht, C. A review of the taxonomy, ethnobotany, chemistry and pharmacology of Sutherlandia frutescens (Fabaceae). *J. Ethnopharmacol*, 2008 119: 620-629.

[330] Johnson, Q; Syce, J; Nell, H; Rudeen, K; Folk, WR. A randomized, double-blind, placebo-controlled trial of Lessertia frutescens in healthy adults. *PLoS Clin. Trials*, 2007 2: e16.

[331] Schwarz, EJ; Reginato, MJ; Shao, D; Krakow, SL; Lazar, MA. Retinoic acid blocks adipogenesis by inhibiting C/EBPbeta-mediated transcription. *Mol. Cell Biol*, 1997 17: 1552-1561.

[332] Elberg, G; Gimble, JM; Tsai, SY. Modulation of the murine peroxisome proliferator-activated receptor gamma 2 promoter activity by CCAAT/enhancer-binding proteins. *J. Biol. Chem*, 2000 275: 27815-27822.

[333] Roy, S; Rink, C; Khanna, S; Phillips, C; Bagchi, D; Bagchi, M; Sen, CK. Body weight and abdominal fat gene expression profile in response to a novel hydroxycitric acid-based dietary supplement. *Gene Expr*, 2004 11: 251-262.

[334] Shara, M; Ohia, SE; Yasmin, T; Zardetto-Smith, A; Kincaid, A; Bagchi, M; Chatterjee, A; Bagchi, D; Stohs, SJ. Dose- and time-dependent effects of a novel (-)-hydroxycitric acid extract on body weight, hepatic and testicular lipid peroxidation, DNA fragmentation and histopathological data over a period of 90 days. *Mol. Cell Biochem*, 2003 254: 339-346.

[335] Kao, YH; Hiipakka, RA; Liao, S. Modulation of endocrine systems and food intake by green tea epigallocatechin gallate. *Endocrinology*, 2000 141: 980-987.

[336] Kovacs, EM; Lejeune, MP; Nijs, I; Westerterp-Plantenga, MS. Effects of green tea on weight maintenance after body-weight loss. *Br. J. Nutr*, 2004 91: 431-437.

[337] Calapai, G; Crupi, A; Firenzuoli, F; Costantino, G; Inferrera, G; Campo, GM; Caputi, AP. Effects of Hypericum perforatum on levels of 5-hydroxytryptamine, noradrenaline and dopamine in the cortex, diencephalon and brainstem of the rat. *J. Pharm. Pharmacol*, 1999 51: 723-8.

[338] Xie, JT; Wang, CZ; Ni, M; Wu, JA; Mehendale, SR; Aung, HH; Foo, A; Yuan, CS. American ginseng berry juice intake reduces blood glucose and body weight in ob/ob mice. *J. Food Sci*, 2007 72: S590-S594.

[339] Moffatt, RJ; Owens, SG. Cessation from cigarette smoking: changes in body weight, body composition, resting metabolism, and energy consumption. *Metabolism*, 1991 40: 465-470.

[340] Perkins, KA; Epstein, LH; Marks, BL; Stiller, RL; Jacob, RG. The effect of nicotine on energy expenditure during light physical activity. *N. Engl. J. Med*, 1989 320: 898-903.

[341] Koch, JE. Delta(9)-THC stimulates food intake in Lewis rats: effects on chow, high-fat and sweet high-fat diets. *Pharmacol. Biochem. Behav*, 2001 68: 539-543.

[342] Koch, JE; Matthews, SM. Delta9-tetrahydrocannabinol stimulates palatable food intake in Lewis rats: effects of peripheral and central administration. *Nutr. Neurosci*, 2001 4: 179-187.

[343] Greenberg, JA; Boozer, CN; Geliebter, A. Coffee, diabetes, and weight control. *Am. J. Clin. Nutr*, 2006 84: 682-693.

INDEX

A

absorption, 10, 11, 16, 18, 19, 20, 35, 36, 38, 54, 58
abstinence, 24
acceleration, 16
accounting, 15
acetylcholine, 23, 60
acid, 2, 12, 14, 15, 16, 20, 27, 35, 36, 37, 38, 40, 49, 50, 51, 52, 57, 58, 60, 66, 70
activation, 48, 56
acute, 13, 21, 23, 25, 30, 67
addiction, 26
adenosine, 15, 23, 29, 35, 59, 60
adipocyte, 19, 23, 37, 55
adipocytes, 16, 21, 25, 36, 58, 67
adiponectin, 7
adipose, 7, 10, 17, 18, 19, 25, 28, 55, 56, 58, 63
adipose tissue, 7, 17, 18, 19, 25, 28, 55, 56, 58, 63
adiposity, 7, 8, 16, 22, 38, 45
administration, 9, 13, 14, 15, 16, 17, 18, 19, 20, 21, 22, 23, 24, 25, 26, 28, 29, 30, 31, 37, 59, 60, 64, 67, 69, 71
adrenaline, 1, 14, 51
adult, 17, 67
adults, ix, 7, 10, 31, 57, 64, 70

adverse event, 14, 28
afferent nerve, 28
Afghanistan, 28
Africa, 26, 27, 28
age, 24, 48
agent, 51, 67, 68
agents, 4, 62
agonist, 21, 35, 59
aid, 21
AIDS, 30, 41, 68
alcohol, 17, 35, 36, 68
alkaloids, 21, 29, 58
alpha, 58
alternative, 4, 11, 17
alters, 7, 15, 23, 24, 25, 63, 64
amine, 65
amines, 26, 65
amphetamine, 1, 4, 8, 26, 65
amygdala, 9
amylase, 16, 35, 36
anabolic, 8
analgesic, 18
animal models, 14
animals, 10, 17, 22, 25, 27, 30, 53
anorexia, ix, 14, 64, 68, 69
anorexia nervosa, 69
antagonist, 30, 47, 68
antagonists, 9, 25, 30, 64
anthropometry, 67
antidepressant, 44, 68
antiobesity, 51, 52, 59

antioxidant, 57
antioxidative activity, 20
anxiety, 4
appetite, 9, 11, 12, 13, 14, 15, 23, 24, 25,
    26, 27, 28, 29, 30, 31, 34, 41, 43, 45,
    48, 49, 50, 51, 60, 61, 62, 63, 64, 65,
    66, 68, 69
Arabia, 28
ARC, 1, 8
arginine, 60
arid, 27
Asia, 14, 19
Asian, 17
Asian cultures, 17
aspartate, 59
ATP, 1, 15, 25, 28, 35, 36, 46, 52, 66
attacks, 44
Australasia, 5
availability, 15, 21

B

back, 29
barbiturates, 68
barrier, 8
basal forebrain, 8, 9
basal metabolic rate, 9, 29, 43, 48, 62
behavior, 46, 47, 60, 62
Beijing, 54
beneficial effect, 12, 13, 19, 21
benefits, 12, 17, 24, 30, 33, 34
benzodiazepine, 69
benzodiazepines, 68
beverages, 23
binding, 7, 25, 63, 70
biological systems, 29
biomarker, 15
biomarkers, 15
biosynthesis, 9
black tea, 19
blocks, 70
blood, 4, 8, 10, 17, 18, 22, 40, 55, 63, 70
blood flow, 10
blood glucose, 8, 17, 18, 55, 70
blood pressure, 4, 10, 40

Blood pressure, 44
blood-brain barrier, 8
BMI, 1, 15, 18, 25, 38, 40, 41
body composition, 10, 21, 33, 63, 67, 70
body fat, 14, 18, 19, 20, 23, 29, 40, 43,
    54, 56, 57, 64
body mass, 18, 20, 27, 58
body mass index, 18
body temperature, 10
body weight, ix, 3, 7, 8, 9, 10, 11, 12,
    13, 14, 15, 16, 17, 18, 19, 20, 21, 22,
    23, 24, 25, 27, 29, 33, 37, 38, 39, 40,
    41, 43, 44, 45, 46, 47, 48, 52, 58, 60,
    62, 63, 64, 66, 67, 69, 70
brain, 8, 15, 23, 26, 27, 30, 31, 36, 43,
    46, 55, 59, 60
brain structure, 23, 31
brainstem, 8, 70
breakdown, 4, 16
bulimia, ix
bulimia nervosa, ix

C

cachexia, 30, 41
caffeine, 19, 20, 23, 24, 33, 34, 38, 55,
    56, 57, 59, 60, 61, 62
caloric intake, 17, 24, 30, 34, 37, 47, 62,
    67
caloric restriction, 43
calorie, 8, 27, 54, 62
cAMP, 24, 29, 36
cancer, 3, 30, 41, 68
cannabinoids, 30, 31, 69
cannabis, 29, 30
carbohydrate, 7, 10, 16, 61
carbohydrates, 8, 10, 15, 16
carcinogenesis, 58
cardiovascular disease, 3, 12, 44
cardiovascular risk, 57
CAS, 58
catabolic, 8
catechins, 18, 19, 20, 35, 36, 38, 54, 55,
    56, 57
catechol, 14

catecholamine, 24, 60
catecholamines, 14, 51, 61
cell, 9, 12, 18
cell line, 12
cell metabolism, 9
central nervous system, 8
channels, 46
chest, 18
chewing, 26, 39, 56, 65
children, ix, 43, 45
China, 16, 18
Chinese medicine, 16, 17, 21
chlorogenic acid, 20, 35, 38, 40, 58
chocolate, 51
cholecystokinin, 45, 49, 50, 66
cholesterol, 14, 15, 22, 29, 54
cholinergic, 23, 35, 47
chromium, 61, 66
chronic disorders, 3
cigarette smoke, 25, 65
cigarette smokers, 25
cigarette smoking, 24, 64, 70
cigarettes, 30, 39
circulation, 20
cis, 49
citalopram, 44
Citrus aurantium, 58
clinical trial, 30, 34
clinical trials, 30, 34
clinically significant, 29
cloning, 45
CNS, 1, 8, 11, 35, 36, 55
cocaine, 8
coffee, 2, 20, 23, 24, 38, 57, 58, 61
cognitive function, 69
cohort, 49, 64
colon, 8
compensation, 13
components, 13, 22, 56
composition, 10, 67
compounds, ix, 20, 26, 27, 28, 29, 30, 33
concentration, 7
confidence, 21
Congress, vi
Connecticut, 51

constraints, 31
consumers, 24, 34
consumption, 10, 12, 13, 15, 18, 19, 21,
    22, 23, 27, 29, 33, 40, 48, 49, 50, 56,
    57, 60, 62, 63, 64, 65, 69, 70
control, 8, 9, 13, 19, 20, 24, 26, 29, 33,
    34, 44, 45, 46, 47, 48, 56, 71
control group, 19, 29
conversion, 24
cooking, 14
coronary heart disease, 49
correlation, 26, 44
cortex, 2, 9, 36, 47, 70
corticotropin, 9, 61
CRH, 1, 9
crystallization, 49
C-terminal, 45
culture, 3
cycles, 24
cyclic AMP, 24, 67

D

de novo, 15, 28
degradation, 24
Demonstration Project, 64
deposits, 23
deprivation, 28, 43
derivatives, 4
desert, 27
detection, 8, 55
diabetes, 3, 16, 27, 44, 71
Diamond, 59
diarrhoea, 4
diet, 10, 12, 22, 27, 28, 37, 38, 49, 51,
    52, 53, 54, 56, 59, 60, 63
dietary, 13, 16, 17, 18, 22, 23, 51, 54,
    67, 70
dietary fat, 18, 67
dieting, 3, 29
diets, 8, 10, 53, 71
differentiation, 19, 36, 55
digestion, 12, 16, 17, 19
dilation, 21
diseases, 17

distribution, 10, 64
DNA, 70
dopamine, 23, 59, 60, 63, 64, 70
dopaminergic, 23, 25
dosing, 13, 27, 30
down-regulation, 55
drinking, 21, 38, 69
drinking water, 38
drug interaction, 44
drugs, 4, 16, 30, 43, 58
drying, 19
duodenum, 8
duration, 21, 25, 27

E

eating, 8, 30, 47, 50
Education, iii
electrochemical detection, 55
emotion, 9
emulsions, 50
endocrine, 8, 9, 70
endocrine system, 9, 70
endurance, 61
energy, ix, 3, 5, 9, 10, 13, 15, 16, 19, 21,
    25, 29, 33, 43, 45, 46, 48, 49, 50, 52,
    56, 57, 60, 61, 63, 65, 66, 70, 71
energy consumption, 10, 15, 70
environment, ix
enzymes, 19, 35
epidemic, ix, 3
epidemiologic studies, 24
epigallocatechin gallate, 19, 55, 70
ERK1, 35
ester, 51
Ethanol, 59
etiology, 43
Europe, 28
evening, 13
evolution, 3
excretion, 15, 24
exercise, 3, 19, 57, 61, 62
exposure, 25
external environment, 3

F

faecal, 4
family, 27, 28, 29, 46
famine, 3, 28
fasting, 8, 47
fat, 4, 7, 11, 12, 13, 14, 15, 16, 18, 19,
    20, 23, 29, 36, 37, 38, 40, 43, 48, 50,
    51, 52, 54, 56, 57, 58, 59, 64, 70, 71
fat soluble, 4
fats, 29, 33
fatty acids, 1, 12, 15, 49, 50
FDA, iii
feedback, 7, 15, 43
feeding, 8, 9, 23, 24, 25, 27, 30, 46, 47,
    48, 50, 53, 59, 60, 65, 69
feelings, 27
fermentation, 19
fish, 29
flavone, 28
flavonoids, 28, 55, 56
flow, 10
fluid, 45
food, 3, 5, 7, 8, 9, 10, 13, 14, 15, 17, 19,
    21, 22, 23, 25, 26, 27, 28, 30, 31, 33,
    34, 37, 38, 39, 40, 41, 43, 45, 46, 47,
    48, 49, 50, 51, 56, 60, 61, 62, 63, 64,
    65, 66, 67, 68, 69, 70, 71
food intake, 5, 7, 8, 9, 13, 14, 15, 17, 19,
    21, 22, 25, 26, 27, 28, 30, 31, 34, 37,
    38, 39, 40, 45, 46, 47, 48, 49, 50, 51,
    61, 62, 63, 64, 65, 66, 67, 68, 69, 70,
    71
forebrain, 47
Fox, ii
fragmentation, 70
fruits, 17, 51
fuel, 10

G

G protein, 46
gastric, 12, 13, 17, 21, 26, 27, 28, 35, 50,
    65

gastrointestinal, 4
gene, 7, 45, 47, 70
gene expression, 70
generation, 25, 31
genes, 7, 15, 35
genotypes, 43
Ghrelin, 7, 45
Gibbs, 45
ginseng, 17, 22, 34, 59, 70
Ginsenoside, 59
GLP-1, 1, 8, 12, 13, 35, 37, 50
glucagon, 8
gluconeogenesis, 20
glucose, 8, 11, 15, 17, 18, 19, 20, 24, 37,
    45, 48, 55, 56, 57, 58, 70
glutamate, 59
glycerol, 1, 9, 47, 69
glycogen, 15, 24
glycoside, 27, 66
glycosides, 28
grains, 29
green tea, 19, 20, 33, 54, 55, 56, 57, 60,
    61, 70
green tea extract, 57
groups, 15, 20, 21
growth, 9, 45, 46, 51
GTE, 2, 19, 20
gums, 19
gut, 8, 13, 35, 49

H

harmful effects, 14
HDL, 15
headache, 14
health, ix, 3, 12, 17, 19, 21, 26, 33
heart, 4, 40, 48, 49, 64
heart disease, 49
heart rate, 4, 48
heat, 9, 25, 48
hedonic, 5, 31, 41, 69
hematological, 67
hepatocytes, 25
herbal, 29, 51, 52, 58
herbal medicine, 29

herbs, 11
Higgs, 69
high fat, 37, 38, 53
high-fat, 51, 52, 54, 56, 59, 71
high-performance liquid
    chromatography, 55
high-risk, 44
hippocampus, 23
HIV, 31, 67, 68
HIV infection, 68
HIV/AIDS, 31
homeostasis, 45
hormone, 1, 7, 8, 12, 45, 46, 47, 48
hormones, 12, 28, 48, 49
horse, 54
human, 3, 11, 12, 17, 40, 41, 43, 45, 48,
    50, 61, 67
human subjects, 61
humans, 3, 8, 9, 14, 15, 16, 17, 18, 19,
    20, 21, 23, 24, 25, 27, 29, 34, 43, 44,
    45, 47, 48, 49, 50, 52, 56, 57, 61, 67
hunting, 28
hydrocarbon, 30
hydrolysis, 16
hypercholesterolemia, 17
hyperglycemia, 51
hyperlipidemia, 3, 17, 53
hypertension, 3
hypertensive, 57
hypotensive, 20, 47, 57
hypothalamic, 8, 9, 22, 25, 28, 35, 36,
    45, 46, 47, 48, 60, 63, 64, 68
hypothalamus, 2, 7, 8, 9, 22, 23, 26, 28,
    29, 35, 46, 47, 60, 66
hypothesis, 14, 31

I

ice, 19
identification, 27
ileum, 8
immune function, 12
in vitro, ix, 11, 12, 16, 20, 49
in vivo, 25, 51, 59, 63
inactivation, 14, 35

India, 28, 29, 66
Indian, 28, 66, 67
indigenous, 14, 27
industrial, 28
inefficiency, 9
infection, 68
inflammation, 52
infusions, 50
ingestion, 25, 27, 56
inhibition, 9, 15, 16, 17, 18, 19, 20, 22,
     54, 56
inhibitor, 4, 16, 52, 54, 58
inhibitors, 57, 61
inhibitory, 18
inhibitory effect, 18
injections, 68
injury, vi
insomnia, 4
insulin, 7, 20, 22, 45, 52, 60
insulin resistance, 52
integration, 8
interaction, 9, 23, 44, 56
interactions, ix, 9, 44, 48, 55, 61
intervention, 23
interviews, 27
intestine, 8, 18
intraocular, 67
intraocular pressure, 67
intraperitoneal, 14
intravenous, 14, 50
intrinsic, 9
irritability, 4
irritable bowel syndrome, 4
isomers, 52

J

JAMA, 51, 64
Japanese, 17, 54
jejunum, 8
Jung, 61

K

King, 44
Korea, 54
Korean, 12, 13, 22, 35, 36, 37, 40, 49, 50

L

LDL, 15, 49, 54
leptin, 7, 9, 15, 22, 36, 37, 45, 46, 63
lesions, 8, 46
lettuce, 26
lifestyle, 3
ligands, 67
linoleic acid, 12, 51
lipase, 4, 17, 18, 21, 22, 25, 35, 36, 38,
     54, 58, 63
lipid, 10, 14, 15, 16, 35, 50, 51, 52, 53,
     70
lipid metabolism, 14, 53
lipid oxidation, 15
lipid peroxidation, 70
lipids, 8, 10, 13, 16, 63
lipolysis, 7, 16, 21, 24, 25, 29, 35, 36,
     58, 63, 67
lipoprotein, 12, 21, 25, 35, 38, 49, 58, 63
liquid chromatography, 55
liver, 20, 51, 53
locomotion, 65
London, 48, 62

M

macronutrients, 3, 16
magnetic, vi
maintenance, 4, 10, 11, 13, 15, 33, 40,
     61, 70
malabsorptive, 16
malaise, 34
males, 18
malondialdehyde, 54
mammals, 7, 47, 48
management, ix, 20, 23, 40, 41, 44, 48,
     50, 52, 53

manipulation, 11, 55
marijuana, 30, 67, 68
market, 4, 13, 22, 26, 28
meals, 3, 10, 14, 24
measures, 29
mediation, 31, 69
medications, 11
Mediterranean, 12, 49
melanin, 8, 46, 47
memory, 68
men, 24, 54, 56, 57, 61, 67
messengers, 26
metabolic, ix, 4, 7, 9, 10, 15, 24, 25, 29,
    43, 48, 49, 53, 55, 57, 61, 62, 63
metabolic rate, 4, 9, 24, 29, 43, 48, 57,
    61, 62, 63
metabolic syndrome, 49, 55
metabolism, 9, 10, 12, 14, 25, 49, 53, 57,
    61, 63, 70
metabolite, 56
metabolites, 15, 57
methylation, 51
mice, 14, 16, 17, 18, 20, 23, 27, 37, 51,
    52, 53, 54, 56, 58, 59, 60, 70
micelle formation, 18
microdialysis, 39, 63
micronutrients, 3
milk, 51
mitochondria, 15, 20
mitochondrial, 28
models, 14, 19
modulation, 56, 59, 60
molecules, ix, 10, 28, 48
monkeys, 67
monoamine, 64
mood, 4, 67, 68
morbidity, ix
mortality, ix
motivation, 3, 5, 9, 31, 60
mouse, 45, 46
mRNA, 63
mucosa, 26

N

NAc, 23, 25, 31, 35, 39
naloxone, 68, 69
Namibia, 27
natural, 12, 31, 51, 52, 66
natural food, 51
nausea, 31
neonates, 9
nerves, 28
nervous system, 1, 2, 45
network, 45
neural network, 45
neural systems, 48
neuroanatomy, 46
neuroendocrine, 12
neuronal systems, 47
neurons, 45, 46, 60
neuropeptide, 8, 47
Neuropeptide Y, 2
neuropeptides, 7, 46
neuroprotective, 55
neurotransmission, 4, 23, 31, 35, 36, 59
neurotransmitters, 23, 25, 31, 63
New York, v, vi, 62, 68
niacin, 66
nicotine, 19, 24, 25, 33, 56, 61, 62, 63,
    64, 65, 71
Nicotine, 24, 25, 35, 39, 41, 63, 64, 65
N-methyl-D-aspartate, 59
non-native, 27
nonsmokers, 62
non-smokers, 24, 25
noradrenaline, 4, 51, 70
Noradrenaline, 2
norepinephrine, 48
normal, 9, 11, 18, 22, 24, 61
nuclei, 9
nucleus, 1, 2, 8, 9, 45, 47, 59, 63, 69
nucleus accumbens, 9, 47, 59, 63, 69
nucleus accumbens (NAc), 9
nutraceutical, 54
nutrient, 11, 19, 27, 65
nutrients, 10, 11
nuts, 12, 49

O

oat, 13, 35, 37, 40
obese, 4, 9, 10, 13, 16, 17, 18, 22, 23,
   24, 27, 37, 43, 45, 46, 50, 52, 53, 54,
   57, 58, 60, 61, 62, 66
obese patients, 4, 43
obesity, ix, 3, 4, 10, 14, 15, 16, 17, 18,
   19, 20, 21, 22, 30, 40, 43, 44, 48, 51,
   53, 54, 55, 56, 57, 58, 59, 60, 64, 67
observations, 30, 64
octapeptide, 45
oil, 12, 13, 16, 35, 37, 40, 49, 50
oils, 12, 33
oleic acid, 12
open-field, 65
opioid, 36, 68, 69
oral, 16, 17, 26, 30, 67, 69
organic, 14
organism, 7, 46
oriental medicine, 17
Orlistat, 4, 44
osteoarthritis, 3
overeating, 69
overnutrition, 10
over-the-counter, 5
overweight, 12, 13, 14, 16, 18, 19, 27,
   29, 49, 50, 52, 57, 58, 64, 67
oxidation, 10, 15, 19, 20, 57
oxidative, 52
oxidative stress, 52

P

pain, 4, 18
palm oil, 13
pancreatic, 17, 18, 22, 35, 36
panic attack, 44
paraventricular, 8
paraventricular nucleus, 8
Parkinson, 55
Parkinson disease, 55
partnership, 28
pathways, 9, 25, 45, 55

patients, 4, 44, 68
peptide, 1, 2, 8, 45
peptides, 8, 26
perception, 23
Peripheral, 12, 22, 35, 36
peroxidation, 70
PFC, 2, 9, 23, 35
pharmacological, 22, 27, 30, 53
pharmacology, 30, 44, 52, 59, 66, 69
pharmacotherapy, 4
phenotypes, 43
phosphodiesterase, 24
phylogenetic, 9
physical activity, 19, 71
physiological, 3, 7, 30
physiology, 43
phytochemicals, ix, 11, 13, 16, 33, 34,
   35, 36, 40
pituitary, 9
pituitary gland, 9
placebo, 13, 14, 18, 19, 21, 26, 27, 29,
   31, 34, 40, 41, 50, 60, 62, 70
plants, ix, 27, 67
plasma, 7, 45, 48, 50, 54
plasma levels, 45
play, 8
pleasure, 69
polyphenols, 53, 55, 57
population, 3, 62
postcessation, 65
postmenopausal, 12, 65
postmenopausal women, 12
powder, 31
preference, 68
press, 23
pressure, 4, 10, 40, 44, 67
Pretoria, 27
prevention, 53, 55
priapism, 21
printing, 55
production, 48, 66
proliferation, 19
promoter, 70
prostaglandin, 61
protein, 2, 7, 12, 25, 47, 48, 63

proteins, 10, 70
psychosis, 44
psychotic, 44
public, 21
public health, 21
PUFAs, 12
pupil, 21
PVN, 2, 8, 68

Q

Quebec, 64

R

raphe, 9
rat, 36, 47, 49, 51, 52, 53, 58, 59, 63, 64, 65, 66, 67, 70
ratings, 30, 31, 39, 41
rats, 9, 14, 17, 22, 23, 26, 27, 31, 39, 45, 46, 51, 52, 53, 54, 56, 57, 58, 59, 60, 61, 62, 63, 64, 65, 66, 68, 69, 71
reactivity, 69
receptor agonist, 9, 59
receptors, ix, 8, 23, 25, 30, 35, 46, 59, 69
reciprocity, 64
regional, 14
regular, 24
regulation, ix, 7, 9, 10, 11, 25, 43, 45, 46, 47, 48, 55, 63, 69
relationship, 24, 45, 47
relationships, 56
relevance, 43
replication, 17
reserves, 21
residential, 61, 67
resistance, 52
respiratory, 14, 29
rewards, 23, 31
risk, 3, 44, 49
risks, 3, 57
rodent, 19, 47, 53
rodents, 9, 14, 16, 21, 22, 23, 25, 37, 54, 55

S

safety, 33, 51, 52, 60
sample, 21, 31
saponin, 17, 22
saponins, 17, 18, 22, 28, 35, 36, 37, 38, 40, 54, 59
saturated fat, 29
saturation, 50
scores, 26
secretion, 7, 12, 17, 27, 35, 50, 65
sedentary, 3
sedentary lifestyle, 3
seed, 49
seeds, 18, 54
self-report, 29
sensation, 13
sensations, 25, 27, 49
sensing, 29, 66
sensitivity, 22
serotonergic, 4, 23, 25
serotonin, 1, 4, 60
serum, 15, 22, 53
services, vi
severity, 64
sex, 24
Short-term, 8, 49, 50, 62
Sibutramine, 4, 44
side effects, 4, 11, 26, 29, 33, 40
signaling, 29
signalling, 46
signals, 7, 8, 10, 43
simulation, 56
sites, 25, 63
skeletal muscle, 19
sleep, 68
small intestine, 17, 50
smoke, 65
smokers, 24, 25, 62, 65, 67, 68
smoking, 24, 25, 39, 41, 62, 63, 64, 70
smoking cessation, 24, 25, 41, 63, 64
SNS, 2, 9, 10, 19, 20
solubility, 54
South Africa, 27
species, 8, 14, 16, 27, 66

specificity, 22
speculation, 31
spinal cord, 47
starvation, 53
stimulant, 62
stomach, 8, 45
storage, 10, 25, 54
stress, 52, 60
striatum, 23
substances, 7, 33, 51
substantia nigra, 9
substrates, 31, 48
sucrose, 31, 35, 68, 69
sugars, 18, 29
sulfate, 58
Sun, 44, 54
supplements, 21, 22
supply, 3
suppression, 11, 15, 25, 47, 56, 60
suppressor, 59
surgery, 16
Surgery, 53, 63, 64
surgical, 16, 21
survival, 3, 7
sweets, 15, 29
sympathetic nervous system, 9, 48
symptoms, 14, 31, 67
synthesis, 14, 15, 67

Tokyo, 53, 54, 60
tolerance, 23, 24, 26, 64
tonic, 9
total cholesterol, 15, 22
total energy, 10
toxic, 14, 21, 52, 58
toxic effect, 21, 58
toxicology, 58
tracers, 47
transcript, 1, 8
transcription, 56, 70
transcription factor, 56
transcription factors, 56
transmission, 23, 35, 60
transport, 15, 55
transportation, 20
transthoracic echocardiography, 43
trial, 29, 31, 44, 49, 50, 51, 53, 57, 60,
    65, 70
tribal, 28
triggers, 9
triglyceride, 24, 25
triglycerides, 2, 12
tumour, 12
type 2 diabetes, 53
type 2 diabetes mellitus, 53
tyrosine, 57

T

targets, ix, 55
taste, 14, 23, 31, 59, 60, 65, 69
taste aversion, 14
taxonomy, 66, 69
tea, 2, 14, 18, 19, 20, 23, 35, 36, 38, 40,
    54, 55, 56, 57
temperature, 10
testis, 52
therapy, 4, 65
thiamin, 60
thyroid, 48
thyrotropin, 9
tissue, 7, 19, 25
tobacco, 24

U

United States, 64
upper respiratory tract, 14
urinary, 15, 24

V

variability, 59
variables, 14, 52
vasopressors, 21
vegetables, 29
Ventral tegmental area, 2
ventricles, 28
vertebrates, 3
visceral adiposity, 52

Vitamin C, ii
Vitamin D, iv
vitamins, 4

W

water, 38
weight changes, 19
weight control, 9, 20, 24, 26, 28, 33, 34,
    44, 56, 71
weight gain, 8, 15, 20, 24, 25, 29, 30, 39,
    41, 62, 63, 64, 65
weight loss, 3, 4, 10, 13, 15, 16, 18, 19,
    20, 21, 24, 25, 27, 29, 30, 33, 34, 40,
41, 45, 47, 48, 51, 57, 61, 62, 64, 66,
    68, 70
weight management, ix, 23, 44, 48, 50,
    52
weight reduction, 15, 57
whole grain, 29
withdrawal, 61
women, 12, 24, 29, 39, 49, 50, 61, 62, 67
wood, 54

Y

Yemen, 26